Osteoporosis

YOUR QUESTIONS ANSWERED

Commissioning Editor: Ellen Green
Project development and management: Fiona Conn
Designer: Jayne Jones, George Ajayi, Keith Kail
Illustrator: Robert Britton

Osteoporosis

YOUR QUESTIONS ANSWERED

John N Fordham

BSc (Hons), MD, FRCP
Consultant Rheumatologist
The James Cook University Hospital, Middlesbrough, UK
Honorary Senior Clinical Lecturer, Newcastle Medical School
Visiting Fellow, Teesside University, School of Health & Social Care

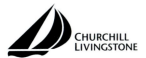
CHURCHILL
LIVINGSTONE

EDINBURGH LONDON NEW YORK OXFORD PHILADELPHIA ST LOUIS SYDNEY TORONTO 2004

CHURCHILL LIVINGSTONE
An imprint of Elsevier Limited

First published 2004

ISBN 0 443 07366 X

British Library Cataloguing in Publication Data
A catalogue record for this book is available from the British Library

Library of Congress Cataloging in Publication Data
A catalog record for this book is available from the Library of Congress

Notice
Medical knowledge is constantly changing. Standard safety precautions must be followed,
but as new research and clinical experience broaden our knowledge, changes in treatment
and drug therapy may become necessary or appropriate. Readers are advised to check the
most current product information provided by the manufacturer of each drug to be
administered to verify the recommended dose, the method and duration of administration,
and contraindications. It is the responsibility of the practitioner, relying on experience and
knowledge of the patient, to determine dosages and the best treatment for each individual
patient. Neither the Publisher nor the author assumes any liability for any injury and/or
damage to persons or property arising from this publication.

 your source for books,
journals and multimedia
in the health sciences
www.elsevierhealth.com

The
publisher's
policy is to use
paper manufactured
from sustainable forests

Printed in China

Contents

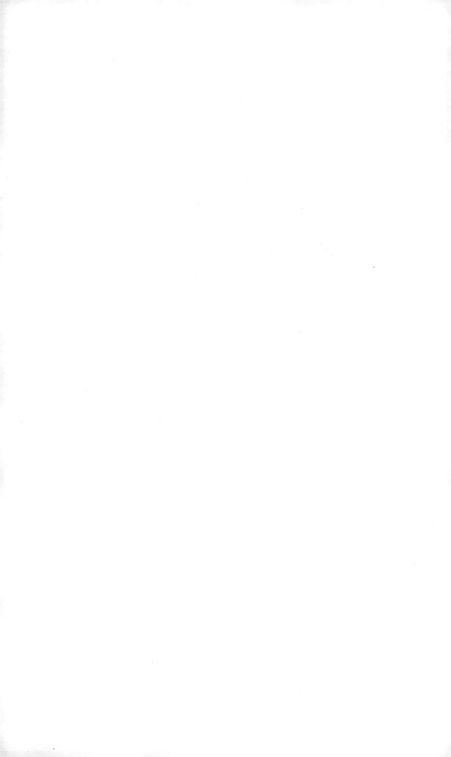

Preface

The burden of osteoporosis in the UK is manifested by over 230 000 fractures per year. The annual cost is £1.7 billion. The condition affects approximately one-third of all women and 1 in 12 men. Fractures carry a risk of death – approximately 20% of patients with hip fractures within a year – and a very high risk of morbidity, particularly for patients with hip and vertebral fractures. Contrasting with these gloomy facts have been the advances in knowledge of the causes of osteoporosis and improvements in methods of detection of people at risk of fractures. It is now possible to offer various preventative and treatment options which have been proven to reduce the risk of fractures. There are an increasing number of novel powerful treatments and formulations being developed. There is therefore, now, little excuse for failing to detect and manage osteoporosis. Since the main burden of osteoporosis is seen in the community, general practitioners/primary care physicians now have a leading role in identifying potential causes.

Patients too have a responsibility to play an active role of their own. This requires a full understanding of the many facets of management. The coming together of diagnostic, therapeutic and self-help components of fracture prevention gives cause for optimism in attempting to reduce the effects of osteoporosis in the future.

J N Fordham

Writing a book is an adventure. To begin with, it is a toy and an amusement. Then it becomes a mistress, then it becomes a master, then it becomes a tyrant. The last phase is that just as you are about to be reconciled to your servitude, you kill the monster, and fling him to the public.

Winston Churchill

ACKNOWLEDGEMENT
I would like to record my thanks to my secretary Miss Angela Coverdale for preparing the manuscript. Throughout the process of writing this book I have been constantly encouraged and supported by my wife Melanie.

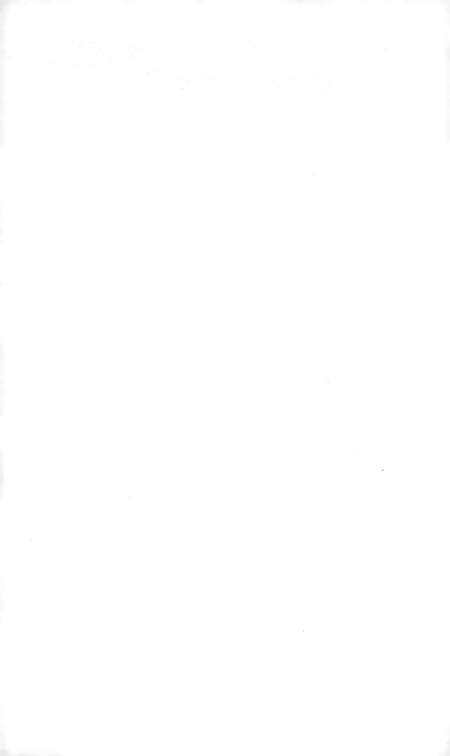

How to use this book

The *Your Questions Answered* series aims to meet the information needs of GPs and other primary care professionals who care for patients with chronic conditions. It is designed to help them work with patients and their families, providing effective, evidence-based care and management.

The books are in an accessible question and answer format, with detailed contents lists at the beginning of every chapter and a complete index to help find specific information. Usually, each topic has an introductory question that sets up the discussion point, followed by a series of questions and answers that examine it in detail. Tables, figures, boxes and icons are used to draw the reader to important points.

ICONS
Icons are used in the book to identify particular types of information:

 highlights information important to clinical practice

 highlights side effect information

PATIENT QUESTIONS
At the end of relevant chapters there are sections of frequently asked patient questions, with easy-to-understand answers aimed at the non-medical reader. These questions are also listed at the end of the book.

Definitions: what is osteoporosis?

1

1.1   What is osteoporosis?

> Osteoporosis has been defined as a systemic, skeletal disease
> characterised by low bone mass and microarchitectural deterioration
> of bone tissue with a consequent increase in bone fragility.

This definition was introduced by an expert panel of the World Health
Organization (WHO) in 1994.[1] It recognises that the condition is silent until
a fracture arises. Bone loss occurs with advancing age and the incidence of
fractures increases with age. Fractures give rise to significant morbidity and
mortality.

The condition occurs three times more frequently in women than in
men, mainly because of the lower peak bone mass attained by women and
because of the hormonal related decline in bone mineral density (BMD)
after the menopause. Because women live longer than men, they are
exposed to a longer period of reduced skeletal bone mass. Women now also
live more than a third of their lives after the menopause. With increasing
ageing of the Western population, the number of postmenopausal women
is increasing. It is anticipated that between 1990 and 2025 the number of
women over 50 years of age will increase by 30–40% in Europe.[2]

1.2   How is low bone mass defined?

The definition of low bone mass (*Table 1.1*) was based on the use of T scores
– standard deviation (SD) measurements of bone mineral density (BMD) or
bone mineral content (BMC) referenced to the young adult mean:

TABLE 1.1 Definitions of osteoporosis/osteopenia (From WHO[1])

Clinical status	Definition
Normal	A value for BMD or BMC not more than 1 standard deviation below the average value of young adults
Low bone mass or osteopenia	A value for BMD or BMC more than 1 standard deviation below the young adult average, but not more than 2.5 standard deviations below
Osteoporosis	A value for BMD or BMC more than 2.5 standard deviations below the young adult average value
Established osteoporosis	A value for BMD or BMC more than 2.5 standard deviations below the young adult average value and the presence of one or more fragility fractures, e.g. hip, wrist or vertebra

$$T = \frac{\text{BMD} - \text{BMD young normal}}{\text{SD young normal}}$$

Measurements are usually taken at the lumbar spine and hip and sometimes the forearm. These measurements are usually taken by using the technique of dual energy X-ray absorptiometry (DXA).

1.3   Why use T scores?

■ Bone mineral density and mass across populations have normal distributions. It is impossible therefore to clearly separate those at risk of fractures from those with low risk. However, the 'setting' of diagnostic thresholds by use of T scores does identify the majority of patients at risk of osteoporotic fractures (*Fig. 1.1*). Thus, T scores define about 30% of postmenopausal women as having osteoporosis at the clinically relevant sites, i.e. hip, forearm and spine. This value is coincident with the prevalence of fractures in the Caucasian female population after 50 years of age.

■ Since bone mineral density declines with age, it follows that the incidence of osteoporosis increases (*Fig. 1.2*). The definition of

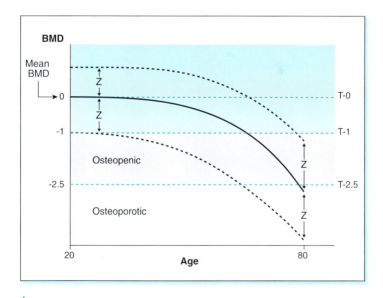

Fig. 1.1 Conceptual representation of T and Z scores.

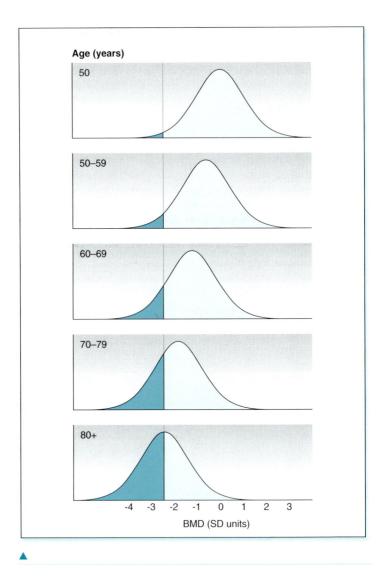

Fig. 1.2 T score thresholds and age. As the population ages, the number of subjects classified as osteoporotic or osteopenic increases. In this case, the incidence of osteoporosis increases to 50% at ages > 80 years. The chances of being found to be osteoporotic increase with the number of sites measured.

osteoporosis by means of bone density or bone mass, ignores the effects of other risk factors for fracture. Bone density however is an important factor in determining fracture risk, and its ease of measurement and the substantive database relating bone density measurements to fracture risk, make this a useful clinical measure for identifying patients at risk of fracture.

1.4   How are T scores used in clinical practice?

The T score system enables clinicians to confirm whether or not patients with risk factors for osteoporosis have this condition. The values should be used in conjunction with other risk factors such as fragility fracture or history of falls to guide patient management. The system was *not* intended to set treatment thresholds. The T score system does have a number of drawbacks which are outlined in *Box 1.1*. However, since its introduction by the WHO it has become broadly accepted in clinical use, not least because most of the drug studies have used T scores to define the populations to be investigated.

BOX 1.1 Drawbacks of T scores

- T scores are of diagnostic value and were not intended as treatment thresholds
- Single cut-off points cannot be interpreted in isolation from the clinical context, in particular in relation to other independent risk factors for fracture
- Discrepancies in T scores occur across different sites within the skeleton and with age
- T scores are not transferable to other technologies (e.g. ultrasound)
- The predictive values for fractures varies across sites and with different DXA devices
- T score definitions have not been derived for all racial groups
- The same T score at different ages has different predictive values (e.g. a T score of –2 at 55 is less likely to be associated with risk of fracture than the same score at 80)

1.5   Why are Z scores sometimes used?

A Z score is the number of standard deviations by which a measurement varies from the mean value of the peer group matched for age, sex and ethnicity. Thus, Z scores are age matched rather than relating to young subjects. The Z score is useful in expressing the relative fracture risk. It is intuitively easier for patients to understand than T scores.

$$Z = \frac{BMD - BMD \text{ age matched subjects}}{SD \text{ age matched subjects}}$$

1.6 What is the importance of osteoporosis?

Using the WHO definition of osteoporosis, i.e. 2.5 standard deviations below the young adult mean, it is possible to assess the size of the problem in the general population. BMD decreases with age and in women particularly after the menopause. It is estimated that 16% of women over the age of 50 will have osteoporosis of the hip. When other sites are measured, the prevalence of osteoporosis in women increases to about 30% (*Table 1.2*).

Osteoporosis is less common in men due to the higher peak bone density and the lower rate of bone loss and because men do not live as long as women. Thus, the skeleton is less exposed to the effect of ageing and the associated medical conditions which 'accumulate' in the older population. The UK lifetime risk of fracture of a 50-year-old white man is 2% for the vertebra and 3% for the hip compared to 11% and 14%, respectively, for women of the same age.

Details about the incidence of the common fractures are found in *Chapter 2*. Hip fractures particularly are associated with a high risk of death. All of the common osteoporotic fractures are associated with significant morbidity as shown in *Table 1.3*. When the pre-fracture state of female patients is taken into account, it is estimated that about 10% with a hip fracture, 4% with vertebral fractures and 2% with forearm fractures become dependent on help in the activities of daily living. The total number of

TABLE 1.2 Prevalence of osteoporosis in Western women (From WHO[1])

Age range (years)	Osteoporosis at any site (%)	Osteoporosis of hip alone (%)
30–39	0	0
40–49	0	0
50–59	14.8	3.9
60–69	21.6	8.0
70–79	38.5	24.5
80+	70.0	47.6
50+	30.3	16.2

TABLE 1.3 Physical and functional impairment associated with osteoporotic fractures in women (From Greendale et al.[3])

	Hip fracture	Spine fracture	Wrist fracture
Movements			
Bend	2.7	3.1	1.2
Lift	1.1	3.4	1.3
Reach	1.5	0.7	1.8
Walk	3.6	2.7	1.6
Climb stairs	2.6	2.2	1.8
Descend stairs	4.1	4.2	2.5
Get into/out of car	1.3	2.1	1.3
Activities			
Put socks on	1.6	1.7	1.1
Cook meals	11.1	6.9	10.2
Shop	4.6	5.2	3.3
Heavy housework	2.8	2.1	1.6

Figures relate to odds of impairment, i.e. likelihood of having the impaired movement or activity following fracture after adjusting for age, body mass index, oestrogen use, visual impairment and reduced mental status.

osteoporotic fractures occurring annually in the UK is £310 000 with a total cost of £1.7 billion.[2]

1.7 What is the fracture threshold?

This is the theoretical concept of a level of bone density below which the incidence of fracture increases significantly. However, an arbitrary bone density level does not clearly differentiate those who have had a fracture from those whom have not. There is an 'overlap' between the fracture and non-fracture groups. One of the reasons for this is that factors other than bone density can influence the risk of fracture, most importantly risk of falling and the physical impact of any fall.

1.8 What is the cost of fractures to an average primary care trust/organisation?

The number of common fractures associated with osteoporosis in the UK was estimated by the National Osteoporosis Society.[4] *Table 1.4* shows that an average primary care organisation (PCO) has 120 hip fractures, 120 wrist fractures and 40 vertebral fractures per year, the total cost being £2.8 million. These include hospital costs, follow-up costs and drug costs. The number of vertebral fractures is underestimated since only a third of these fractures come to medical attention.

TABLE 1.4 Cost of osteoporotic fractures in primary care organisations (PCO) (From National Osteoporosis Society[4])

Type of fracture	No. of fractures per PCO (100 000 patients)	Acute costs (£) per fracture	Per PCO (£)	Total costs (£)* per fracture	Per PCO (£)
Hip	120	5300	636 000	21 500	2 580 000
Wrist	120	500	60 000	500	60 000
Vertebral (clinically diagnosed)	40	500	20 000	500	20 000
Other	100	1400	140 000	1400	140 600
Total cost			856 000		2 800 600

* Includes social care and long stay hospital costs, follow-up costs and drug costs.

Apart from the costs, the impact of fractures on the quality of life of patients is considerable. Inevitably, wrist and hip fractures are initially managed in secondary care. However, it is clear that the implications of fractures are often overlooked by medical practitioners in both primary and secondary care. The majority of such patients are not assessed for possible secondary osteoporosis or bone densitometry. This missed opportunity reflects the absence of systems in place to identify patients who have had fractures. Currently detection and management of osteoporosis tends to be opportunistic rather than planned and coordination between secondary and primary care in the postfracture management of such patients is often lacking.

1.9 How is osteoporosis currently managed in general practice?

Within the UK the National Osteoporosis Society conducted a survey of osteoporosis management in primary care in 1999.[5] The study was taken from a sample of over 1000 general practitioners (GPs). The data were collected by telephone interview and the results from 200 GPs were studied. This showed that over the period from 1994 to 1999 access to DXA had increased, with 36% of GPs being able to use such facilities. However, access was often via consultant referral rather than an open access system. Most GPs accessed DXA using the Royal College of Physicians (RCP) guidelines.[6]

Almost a quarter (24%) of GPs reported that they referred *all* menopausal women for DXA (*Table 1.5*). This suggested that screening for osteoporosis was appropriate, whereas current best practice is for selective case finding using the RCP guidelines to identify patients at risk. The

TABLE 1.5 Patients who should be referred for bone densitometry (From National Osteoporosis Society survey of 1999[5])

Patient group	Frequency of referral (%)
All menopausal women	24
All women 50+	13
All men and women 50+	5
Anyone with a minimal trauma fracture	82
Patients prescribed corticosteroids	76
Early menopause	80
Family history	81

TABLE 1.6 Prescribing for osteoporosis in general practice (From National Osteoporosis Society survey of 1999[5])

Therapeutic agent	Frequency of prescribing (%)				
	Always	Often	Sometimes	Seldom	Never
Calcium alone	2	6	32	23	38
Calcium and vitamin D	8	30	42	12	10
HRT	4	52	33	7	6
Etidronate	4	40	40	12	5
Alendronate	1	12	42	21	25
Raloxifene	0	2	14	18	87
Analgesia	9	34	42	10	6

primacy of DXA as a diagnostic tool was accepted with only 8% using ultrasound-based techniques and 12% using quantitative computed tomography (QCT). A surprising finding was the use of bone markers with 27% reporting having used this technique. This suggests some misunderstandings about the role of bone markers in the diagnosis and management of osteoporosis.

Lifestyle advice was offered by the majority of GPs. Drug management showed considerable variations in therapy with 64% of women who had had an early menopause being treated prophylactically, with 48% prescribing for corticosteroid users, 13% for the housebound elderly and 24% if there was a family history of fracture (*Table 1.6*).

In synopsis, there was awareness by GPs of the importance of identifying those at risk of osteoporosis, treating them and paying attention to adverse lifestyle factors. Management was usually directed at those who had had a fracture, with some GPs having difficulty in accessing bone densitometry. Use of guidelines was variable (*Table 1.7*) and these were more likely to be taken up when they were locally generated.

TABLE 1.7 Use of guidelines (From National Osteoporosis Society survey of 1999[5])

Guideline	Had seen (unprompted) (%)	Had seen (prompted) (%)	Used (%)	Actively adopted (%)
NOS corticosteroid guides	10	35	22	14
DOH guide	3	31	11	6
RCP guidelines	1	13	3	2
Local guidelines	30	43	33	29
Others	17	16	N/A	N/A
None	68	37	15	21

DOH, Department of Health; NOS, National Osteoporosis Society; RCP, Royal College of Physicians.

1.10 What is the potential role of primary care in the management of osteoporosis?

In common with other chronic diseases such as ischaemic heart disease and diabetes, primary care physicians/general practitioners (GPs) have the primary role in the detection and management of osteoporosis. The potential tasks within this role are:

- identify those at risk
- establish the diagnosis
- investigate as needed
- initiate treatment
- refer to specialists of particular patient groups, such as children and men
- monitor treatment and compliance.

GPs are in an ideal position to identify patients at risk, particularly since about 70% of patients consult their GPs each year and 90% will consult them over a 5-year period. GPs are experienced in disease detection and management with primary and secondary management being a part of their role.[7]

1.11 What tools do the primary care team have at their disposal?

- Validated risk factors for osteoporosis have been identified so that subjects at risk can be identified.
- Diagnostic facilities are now commonly available, particularly DXA, to confirm the diagnosis of osteoporosis.
- There are increasing number of drugs for both prevention and the treatment of osteoporosis.

■ Modification of lifestyle may contribute to a reduction in fracture risk.
■ Guidelines are available which can be used to promote good practice.[6, 8–10]

 PATIENT QUESTIONS

1.12   What is osteoporosis?

Osteoporosis is a condition of thinning of bone with loss of bone strength; susceptibility to fracture of bone is normal with age, especially in women after middle age. In osteoporosis the extent of the bone loss is greater than average. Because women have less bone than men to start with and since they have additional loss of bone after the menopause, the risk of osteoporosis is much greater for women than for men. In the UK 1 in 3 women and 1 in 12 men have osteoporosis. The fractures commonly associated with osteoporosis occur at the wrist, spine and hip. Because of the increasing age of the population, there is an increasing risk of fracture in old age.

1.13   Why is osteoporosis sometimes called the 'silent epidemic'?

This is because until a fracture occurs, patients are usually unaware that they have osteoporosis. Since bone loss itself it not associated with pain, it is for many patients the unexpected fracture that first suggests the diagnosis of osteoporosis. Often by the time a fracture has occurred a significant amount of bone thinning has taken place. Therefore the emphasis should be on detecting and treating the condition *before* fractures occur.

1.14   How is osteoporosis confirmed?

Patients with risk factors for osteoporosis may have their bone density measured in order to define the amount of bone present. The internationally agreed methodology uses measurements related to the peak bone mass in young adults as a reference point. Using this, individuals can be assessed for risk of fracture. This system employs the so-called T score. Measurements are usually undertaken by means of dual energy X-ray absorptiometry (DXA).

1.15   Why is it important that my GP finds out whether I have osteoporosis?

Osteoporosis is a common condition in the general population. The consequences of end stage osteoporosis – fracture – are potentially serious. For example hip fractures are associated with a high incidence of death (20% in the first year). The cause of death is not the fracture itself, but rather the complications relating to the surgical management of the fracture, compounded by coexistent general health problems and the frailty of patients which increase the chance of infections, bedsores, blood clots, etc. Those who survive fractures may have great difficulty in returning to their previous capabilities and the quality of their life may suffer. Thus, many patients who are just on the 'cusp' of managing independently at home before fracture may move into nursing or residential homes after a fracture.

Within the UK a considerable amount of National Health Service resources are occupied in dealing with the consequences of fractures, with up to 20% of orthopaedic beds being occupied by such patients. The total cost is estimated at £1.7 billion.

We know a lot about the risk factors for osteoporosis so it is often possible to identify those at risk before a fracture occurs. The emphasis in general practice is to have systems to identify those at risk and direct investigation and treatment to them. Techniques to measure bone density are increasingly available to GPs to enable them to confirm osteoporosis and to make decisions about the treatment of their patients. It should thus be possible to identify those at risk and confirm or refute their risk of fracture, and in this way to intervene to reduce the risk of fracture in later life.

1.16 How is osteoporosis managed in general practice?

At present the evidence of current management of osteoporosis in general practice shows this to be largely unplanned and reactive rather than planned and proactive with relatively few practices having systems in place to identify those at risk. Often those that do have a fracture – be that wrist, spine or hip – are not routinely assessed for osteoporosis. There is a similar lack of awareness of the importance of detecting osteoporosis in those patients who have their fractures treated in hospitals.

GPs have responsibilities for the health of the population they serve and are ideally placed to adopt systems to identify those at risk and to further manage those with osteoporosis. They have an increasing armoury of interventions (lifestyle, drugs and others) which may reduce the risk of fractures in the population. Guidelines have been published to promote good practice and are widely available to help in the setting up of systems to help identify those at risk of osteoporosis and as guides to treatment.

1.17 How can I find out more about osteoporosis?

The National Osteoporosis Society (NOS) is the major UK charity supporting patients with osteoporosis, providing practical help in the form of a telephone helpline, local support groups, newsletters, publications of allied literature, support to medical research, and is a strong lobbyist for improvement of bone health in the UK. Contact details for the NOS can be found in *Appendix 1*.

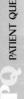

PATIENT QUESTIONS

Epidemiology: how common is osteoporosis?

2

2.1   What is the definition of an osteoporotic fracture?

Although there is no uniformly agreed definition for osteoporotic fractures, in practice, these are usually defined as low impact/low energy fractures, often occurring from a standing height. Fractures of the forearm, spine and hip are usually considered in this category. They share a number of common features: a higher incidence in women; an increased incidence with age; and a tendency to occur at sites of high trabecular bone content.

It is important however to note that other fractures such as those of the humerus, pelvis, ribs and tibia are also associated with low bone mineral density. Thus, the exclusion of such fractures from the definition will lead to an underestimate of the true incidence and costs of osteoporotic fractures.

2.2   What is the incidence of the common osteoporosis-related fractures?

Fractures of the forearm, spine and hip increase with age. In women, up to the age of 35, there is an increased incidence above men. The risk of fractures increases after the menopause, but differentially, i.e. the first peak of fracture rate occurs in the forearm in the first two decades after the menopause and spinal fractures increase in incidence subsequently, reaching a peak in the seventh and eighth decades in women. Lastly, there is an increase in the incidence of hip fractures, climbing exponentially and reaching a maximum in the last two decades of life. There is also a second peak in wrist fracture in extreme old age (*Fig. 2.1*).

A study of Australian women[2] showed an age-specific increase in sustaining fractures from 1.9% in women less than 55 to 49.1% in women aged 89 and over. This study also showed that the risk of subsequent fracture increased such that 2.8% had a further fracture in the first 5 years after the age of 50 and 61.6% after the age of 89 (*Fig. 2.2*).

The likelihood of hospital admission increases with age and with the particular fracture concerned. Thus, nearly all hip fractures result in hospitalisation, but only a third of patients with a vertebral fracture come to clinical attention and only a minority of these are admitted. Similarly, a very small proportion of patients with forearm fractures are admitted, usually the very elderly.

For men, the age and presentation of fractures and the order of fracture presentation differs from women. Thus, significant increases in fracture rates occur only after about 75, vertebral fractures occurring earlier than forearm fractures. The 'profile' of forearm fractures is spread over a longer

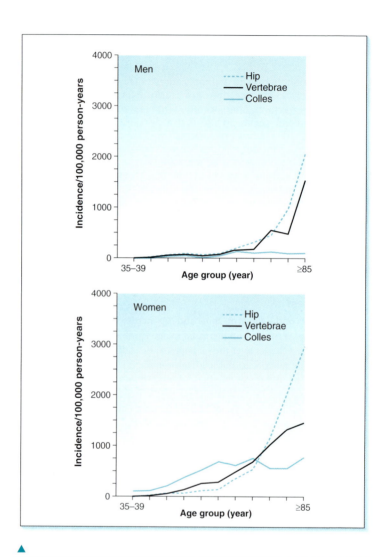

Fig. 2.1 Fractures as a function of age. 5–10 year age shift in age-specific incidence of clinical vertebral and hip fractures. (From Cooper & Melton[1])

age range than in women. There is a similar increase in both hip and spinal fractures in men as is seen in women, but the 'upturn' in men is seen about 10 years after that in women.

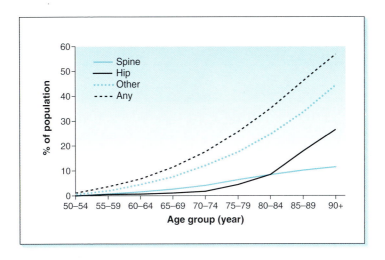

Fig. 2.2 Age-specific proportion of women alive who have sustained at least one osteoporotic fracture since age 50 years. (From Doherty et al.[2])

As with the common osteoporosis-related fractures, fractures at other sites such as the pelvis and upper humerus also increase with age.

Overall, the relative risk of mortality doubles following a clinical fracture. This is mainly due to the increased mortality after hip and spinal fractures, the relative risk of death for spinal and hip fracture patients being nine- and sixfold greater, respectively (*Fig. 2.3*).

2.3   Why are there differences in the incidence of fractures between men and women?

Peak bone mass in men is on average 15% greater than in women. Thus, men have a larger bone 'bank', prior to the age-related decline in bone density that occurs in the ageing skeleton. Secondly, there is no accelerated rate of bone loss seen in men as there is in women after the menopause. This is not to deny the fact that there is a gradual decline in bone mass in ageing men. However, this decline is slower and over a longer period of time compared to the relatively accelerated fall which occurs in women after the menopause.

The differences in the order and incidence of fractures between the sexes may also reflect differential physical activity and occupational differences. Studies have shown that men are more likely to be physically active in later

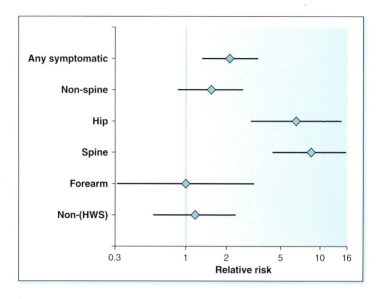

Fig. 2.3 Risk of mortality following clinical fractures. Non-(HWS), non-wrist, non-hip, non-spine. (From Cauley et al.[3])

life than women, which may have an effect on bone density, muscular bulk and reducing the liability to falls. Similarly, the increase in incidence of vertebral fractures seen in men in middle life may reflect the physical nature of occupations that men may undertake.

The lifetime loss of bone between the sexes has been estimated as 45% of trabecular bone and 15% of cortical bone for men compared with 50% and 30% respectively for women. The pathological changes in bone differ between men and women. Cortical bone accretion continues in ageing men and, although there is loss of cancellous bone, the trabecular structure tends to be maintained, albeit with narrower trabeculae. Thus, bone connectivity is relatively retained in men compared with women.

Other differences between the sexes in relation to the incidence of fractures and the type of fracture may be attributable to a differential importance of risk factors between the sexes. Thus alcohol excess is more common in men than in women. The difference in hip fracture incidence between men and women is likely to be related to increased prevalence of disability in women which is double that for men at any age.

HIP FRACTURE

2.4   How do hip fractures occur?

Most hip fractures occur after a fall from a standing height. Usually this happens indoors. The risk of falling increases with age and is greater in women. In England, the average age of presentation is 75.[4] There is a seasonal variation in hip fractures with an increased risk during the winter months although relatively few occur out of doors. The seasonal variation may be related to differences in vitamin D metabolism and the effects of hypothermia on neuromuscular function.

There is a continuing debate as to whether spontaneous fractures occur and whether a fall comes as a consequence of this. Most fractures however appear to follow a direct injury to the hip and the risk of fracture is less if the fall is not directly onto the hip.[5] Some patients report pain on weight bearing for several days prior to the fracture suggesting that a stress fracture may be evolving over this time.

Most hip fractures occur in elderly, infirm patients with coexistent medical conditions which increase the risk of falls (e.g. hypotension, unsteadiness, poor vision). The risk of fracture increases if the impact forces are high as in those who have a low body mass index (BMI) or who have a poor protective response, i.e. ability to brace themselves against a fall. Those who fall sideways as opposed to forwards also expose the trochanter to a greater direct force. Factors which adversely affect bone strength – such as low bone density or geometric factors such as a long neck of femur (particularly associated with Scandinavian populations) – will also increase the likelihood of fracture. Conditions which adversely influence bone quality such as coexistent osteomalacia may also be present in elderly, infirm housebound subjects (*Table 2.1*).

TABLE 2.1 Major risk factors for hip fracture

Secondary causes of osteoporosis	Conditions associated with falls
Thyroidectomy	Hemiparesis
Gastric surgery	Parkinson's disease
Hypogonadism	Dementia
Anticonvulsants	Visual impairment
Alcoholism	Alcoholism
Oral corticosteroids	Drugs, e.g. benzodiazepines
	Hypotension
	Arthritis

2.5   What are the different types of hip fracture?

There are two main groups: cervical and intertrochanteric (*Fig. 2.4*). The type of fracture sustained reflects the type of fall, and biomechanical factors include the amount of cushioning (i.e. subcutaneous fat overlying the hip)

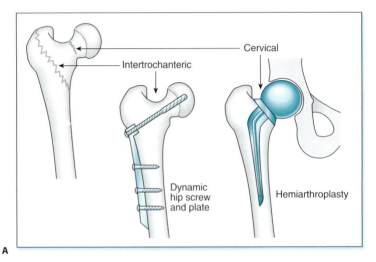

A

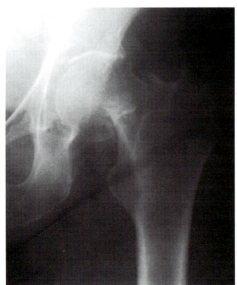

B

Fig. 2.4 A, Types of hip fracture; **B**, cervical hip fracture; **C**, inter-trochanteric hip fracture.

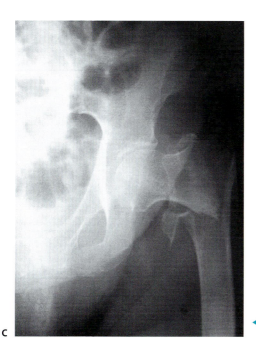

C

◀ **Fig. 2.4 Contd**

as well as the neuromuscular response of the patient to the fall. Intertrochanteric hip fractures are more strongly associated with osteoporosis than cervical fractures, and it is this group which has largely contributed to the increased incidence of hip fractures in Western countries. Patients with intertrochanteric hip fractures tend to be older than those sustaining cervical fractures.

2.6 What is the usual surgical treatment for these two types of fracture?

The type of surgical procedure undertaken reflects the vascularity of the femoral head. Therefore, displaced cervical fractures, which are associated with an increased incidence of avascular necrosis, are usually treated by replacement hemiarthroplasty. Those which are undisplaced and where the femoral head is thought to be viable, are often fixed in situ. A proportion of these will develop avascular necrosis and require revision to total joint arthroplasty or hemiarthroplasty. Intertrochanteric fractures are normally reduced and fixed with a dynamic hip screw (DHS) and plate (*Fig. 2.5*). Alternatively traction may be used, but this, with attendant prolonged bed rest, increases both the risk of complications and the likelihood of prolonged hospitalisation.

2.7 What are the complications of hip fracture?

A hip fracture is the most severe form of osteoporosis-related fracture in terms of morbidity and mortality.[6] The variability is partly a reflection of the combination of premorbid conditions which give rise to increased risk of complications in the elderly. The increased mortality is maximal shortly after the fracture, standardised mortality rates being 2.7 during the first year after fracture.[7] Causes of death include pneumonia, thrombotic events,

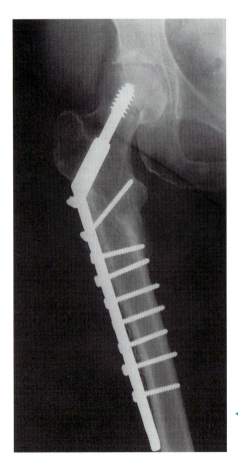

Fig. 2.5 Intertrochanteric fracture with dynamic hip screw.

septicaemia and heart failure. The average length of stay in hospital in most Western countries is 30 days.[8]

2.8 What are the mortality rates of patients with hip fracture?

Mortality rates of up to 20% occur over the first 6–12 months following fracture. Overall, the 5-year survival rate is 0.82.[9] Functional impairment is considerable in terms of performance of activities of daily living. Such disabilities are followed by liability to loss of independence and increased use of nursing homes and care agencies.

2.9 Which factors increase the risk of mortality and morbidity following hip fracture?

Delayed surgery has a profound effect on fracture morbidity. The National Confidential Enquiry into perioperative deaths in the UK in 1993–1994 found that 75% of deaths in orthopaedics occur following hip fracture surgery. It appears that only a minority of operations were performed by consultants.[10] A more recent report has shown that most operations are carried out by specialist registrars, staff grade doctors and with junior anaesthetists.[11] Surgical complications occurred in 30% of cases of which 21% were non-union of the fracture and 12% avascular necrosis. Postoperative complications include urinary infections, pressure sores, pneumonia and deep vein thrombosis – prophylactic low dose heparin and aspirin reduce the risk of thrombosis.[12]

Patients who have hip fractures are usually elderly and have coexistent morbidity, are often confused and have a low BMI. These factors, together with the catabolic reaction to the injury, compounded in many cases by poor postoperative nutrition including protein deficiency, contribute to the increased risk of complications. Supplemental enteral feeding may benefit such patients.

Active rehabilitation may shorten the period of inpatient care. Although the concept of orthogeriatric units is widely held to be a method for improving outcome following hip fracture their validity is unproven.

2.10 What are the effects of hip fracture on the quality of life for patients?

Studies have shown that patients who have survived hip fracture show an increased dependency on walking aids. Only 40% who had been independently mobile before fracture regain their independence. Those who had used a walking stick prior to the fracture were more likely to need a walking frame subsequently.[6] About one-third of women become dependent after hip fracture and of these two-thirds require nursing home care[13] (*Table 2.2*).

TABLE 2.2 Probability of outcome after hip fracture according to functional status before fracture (From Chrischilles et al.[13])

Status before fracture	Independent	Dependent	Nursing home
Independent	0.74	0.18	0.08
Dependent		0.50	0.50
Nursing home			1.0

2.11 What are the particular risk factors for hip fracture?

The Study of Osteoporotic Fractures in North America[14] showed that age, anticonvulsant use, previous hyperthyroidism and maternal history of fracture were important risk factors for hip fractures. Additionally, physical indices such as resting pulse rate above 80 beats per minute, inability to rise from a chair or being mobile for less than 4 hours per day were also independent risk factors (*Table 2.3*).

Others factors predisposing to falls included cerebrovascular accident (CVA), parkinsonism, dementia, visual impairment, use of anxiolytic drugs or alcohol excess. A subsequent reanalysis of these risk factors reduced the number from 16 to 4: low body weight, family history, previous fracture and current smoker.[15]

2.12 What is the relative importance of bone mineral density as opposed to falls in the causation of hip fracture?

The major determinants of fracture are risk of falls, impact force and bone strength. As can be seen from *Table 2.4*, a fall to the side is of more importance than low bone mineral density. Falls to the side and direct hip impact are independent risk factors for fracture both in the community and in nursing homes. Low BMI and reduced physical activity are also associated with increased risk of fractures. This research would suggest that targeting elderly subjects who have such risk factors, might be an appropriate prevention strategy.[16]

2.13 Is there a difference in mortality between the sexes after hip fracture?

The absolute number of men with hip fracture is lower than the number of women (partly reflecting the fact that there are fewer older men than women); about 30% of hip fractures worldwide occur in men. There is an increased mortality in men – the sex of the individual is one of the strongest predictors of death.[17] The increased mortality after hip fracture in men continues over 2 years following fracture whereas women have increased mortality over only the first few months after hip fracture.

TABLE 2.3 Risk factors for hip fracture in Caucasian women (From Cummings et al.[14])

Independent factors	Relative risk (95% confidence interval)	
	Base model	Add fractures and bone density
Age (per 5 years)	1.5 (1.3–1.7)	1.4 (1.2–1.6)
Maternal history of hip fracture (versus none)	2.0 (1.4–2.9)	1.8 (1.2–2.7)
Increase in weight since the age of 25 years (per 20%)	0.6 (0.5–0.7)	0.8 (0.6–0.9)
Height at the age of 25 years (per 6 cm)	1.2 (1.1–1.4)	1.3 (1.1–1.5)
Self-rated health (per 1-point decrease)	1.7 (1.3–2.2)	1.6 (1.2–2.1)
Previous hyperthyroidism (versus none)	1.8 (1.2–2.6)	1.7 (1.2–2.5)
Current use of long acting benzodiazepines (versus no current use)	1.6 (1.1–2.4)	1.6 (1.1–2.4)
Current use of anticonvulsant drugs (versus no current use)	2.8 (1.2–6.3)	2.0 (0.8–4.9)
Current caffeine intake (per 190 mg/day)	1.3 (1.0–1.5)	1.2 (1.0–1.5)
Walking for exercise (versus not doing so)	0.7 (0.5–0.9)	0.7 (0.5–1.0)
On feet ≤ 4 hours/day (versus > 4 hours/day)	1.7 (1.2–2.4)	1.7 (1.2–2.4)
Inability to rise from a chair without the help of arms (versus no inability)	2.1 (1.3–3.2)	1.7 (1.1–2.7)
Lowest quartile for distance depth perception (versus other three)	1.5 (1.1–2.0)	1.4 (1.0–1.9)
Low-frequency contrast sensitivity (per 1 SD decrease)	1.2 (1.0–1.5)	1.2 (1.0–1.5)
Resting pulse > 80 beats/minute (versus ≤ 80)	1.8 (1.3–2.5)	1.7 (1.2–2.4)
Any fracture since the age of 50 years (versus none)	–	1.5 (1.1–2.0)
Calcaneal bone density (per 1 SD decrease)	–	1.6 (1.3–1.9)

TABLE 2.4 Factors influencing risk of hip fracture

Factor	Relative risk
Fall to the side	2.5
Decrease of 1 standard deviation BMD	2.0
Direct hip impact	4.9
Previous CVA	2.9
Reduced functional mobility of 1 standard deviation	2.0
BMD reduction of 1 standard deviation	1.8

BMD, bone mineral density; CVA, cerebrovascular accident.

2.14 What are the reasons for the higher mortality after hip fracture in men?

There are several candidates for the increased mortality in men. These include coexistent general medical conditions, reduced cognitive function, poor functional status and institutionalisation. Morbidity relating to hip fracture is also significantly greater in men and studies from the Mayo Clinic showed that following hip fracture only 21% of men were living independently and 23% lived in some form of institution (of which only one in five was independently mobile and 12% were completely immobile).[18]

2.15 What are the differences in hip fracture incidence rates between races and countries?

There is a striking geographical variation in the incidence of hip fractures between Northern Europe and Southern Mediterranean countries. The highest rates occur in Scandinavian countries. Intermediate rates of incidence are seen in Asian countries and the lowest overall rate in Afro-Caribbean populations[19] *(Table 2.5)*. In the latter, the rates in men and women approach equality. Studies in the USA have also shown significant north/south gradients of risk, with socio-economic deprivation, reduced sunlight exposure and soft water being associated with greatest risk as well as racial origin. In a large sample from the United States, 17% of postmenopausal Caucasian women had osteoporosis of the hip compared to 12% of Hispanic women and 8% of Afro-American women. These differences may account for the differential incidence of fractures between these groups. Other factors such as body composition and relative retention of muscle and fat in Afro-Caribbean women may also be important in determining the incidence of fractures.

The incidence of hip fractures is rising in the Far East. In Hong Kong the incidence of hip fractures has doubled over the last 30 years. The evidence suggests that the increase is proportional to the economic development. In short, the more wealthy the population the higher the risk of hip fractures.

It is predicted that by the year 2050 more than half of all hip fractures in the world will occur in Asia.

2.16 What are the secular trends in hip fracture incidence?

The incidence of fractures in Western countries has been increasing. However, the recent evidence would suggest that the rate of incline is slowing, as confirmed in studies from Sweden, Switzerland and Italy. A large UK study between 1968 and 1986 showed a very marked increase in hip fracture rate over the period 1968–1980 with a subsequent reduction.[20]

TABLE 2.5 Age-adjusted rates[a] of hip fracture per 100 000 population for females, males and total (both age and gender adjusted), by ethnic group and year of study (Reprinted from Marcus et al[19])

Ethnic group	Site [Ref.]	Years of study	Female	Male	Total	Female: Male
Blacks	USA	1986–1989	214	179	200	1.2
	Maryland, USA	1979–1988	345	191	283	1.8
	USA	1984–1985	344	235	300	1.5
	California, USA	1983–1984	241	153	202	1.6
	Texas, USA	1980	243	13	141	18.7
	USA	1974–1979	174	108	137	1.6
	Johannesburg, SA	1950–1964	26	20	23	1.3
Hispanics[b]	California, USA	1983–1984	219	97	165	2.3
	Texas, USA	1980	305	128	227	2.4
Asians	Tottori, Japan	1986–1987	227	79	163	2.9
	Hong Kong	1985	389	196	304	2.0
	Okinawa, Japan	1984–1985	325	86	219	3.8
	California, USA	1983–1984	383	116	265	3.3
	Hawaii, USA	1979–1981	224	66	153	3.4
	New Zealand	1973–1976	212	121	172	1.8
	Hong Kong	1965–1967	179	113	150	1.6
	Singapore	1955–1962	83	111	95	0.7
Caucasians[c]	USA	1986–1989	968	396	738	2.4
	Maryland, USA	1979–1988	950	358	712	2.7
	Sweden	1985	714	268	517	2.7
	USA	1984–1985	845	350	645	2.4
	Canada	1976–1985	788	307	595	2.6
	California, USA	1983–1984	617	215	439	2.9
	Norway	1983–1984	737	298	543	2.5
	Oxford, England	1983	603	114	392	5.3
	USA	1970–1983	705	244	506	2.9
	Minnesota, USA	1978–1982	613	285	468	2.2
	Hawaii, USA	1979–1981	645	205	451	3.1
	Alicante, Spain	1974–1984	90	57	75	1.6
	Sweden	1972–1981	714	319	540	2.2
	Sweden	1972–1981	730	581	664	1.3
	Finland	1980	432	199	329	2.2
	Dundee, Scotland	1980	550	—	—	—
	Sweden	1980	984	338	705	2.9
	Texas, USA	1980	593	223	430	2.7
	Oslo, Norway	1978–1979	850	329	620	2.6
	Edin, Scotland	1978–1979	529	174	376	3.0
	USA	1974–1979	422	151	285	2.8
	Funen, Denmark	1973–1979	4863	200	2804	24.3

TABLE 2.5 Age-adjusted rates[a] of hip fracture per 100 000 population for females, males and total (both age and gender adjusted), by ethnic group and year of study (Reprinted from Marcus et al,[19] with permission from Elsevier)—Contd

Ethnic group	Site [Ref.]	Years of study	Female	Male	Total	Female: Male
	Yorkshire, UK	1973–1977	310	102	218	3.0
	New Zealand	1973–1976	466	139	321	3.4
	Rochester, USA	1965–1974	559	191	396	2.9
	Finland	1970	377	142	273	2.7
	Kuopio, Finland	1968	280	107	204	2.6
	Jerusalem, Israel	1957–1966	355	168	272	2.1
	Malmo, Sweden	1950–1960	468	153	329	3.1

[a]Rates were age and gender adjusted to the 1990 US non-Hispanic Caucasian population; [b]Hispanic Caucasians; [c]Non-Hispanic Caucasians.

VERTEBRAL FRACTURE

2.17 How do vertebral fractures present?

Most vertebral fractures come to light as X-ray findings in patients investigated because of spinal deformity, height loss or back pain. Only about one-third of patients with vertebral fractures come to medical attention. Those that do often give a history of onset of pain after minimal trauma such as twisting movements, coughing, straining or sneezing. Such presentations are commonest in the elderly, frail group. At the other end of the age range, severe trauma such as that due to a road traffic accident may cause vertebral fractures, particularly in younger men. Overall, only about 2% of patients with vertebral fractures are admitted to hospital.[21]

2.18 What are the consequences of vertebral fracture?

■ *Pain* – Those presenting with acute vertebral fractures usually describe central spinal pain characteristically in the mid-dorsal or thoracolumbar areas often with radicular symptoms (e.g. girdle-like pain radiating to the anterior chest or lower abdomen). Characteristically twisting movements such as turning over in bed are exquisitely painful. Most patients take to their bed. Occasionally vertebral fractures may present with true radicular signs and even the cauda equina syndrome. In some patients, ileus and abdominal distension may occur, possibly due to retroperitoneal haemorrhage at the lower thoracic and lumbar sites. Bony tenderness can usually be elicited at the affected level by pressure or percussion over the fracture site. There is often paravertebral muscular spasm with associated muscular tenderness. The pain of a first fracture usually eases over a period of 6–7 weeks.

■ *Chronic pain* – Multiple fractures are associated with increased incidence of chronic pain. This may be due to increased angulation (e.g. kyphosis of the dorsal spine with resultant hyperextension of the neck and increased cervical muscular tension). Other possible mechanisms include facetal osteoarthritis, muscular pain emanating from the paraspinal musculature and radicular pain. Typically chronic spinal pain is characterised by worsening with standing, stooping or lifting.

■ *Spinal deformity* – The risk of kyphosis increases with a number of vertebral fractures. This characteristically gives rise to a smooth mid-dorsal hump, the consequences of which include reduced vital capacity, abutment of the ribs against the pelvic brim, abdominal distension and hiatus hernia.

■ *Depression* – This is common in the context of chronic pain, skeletal deformity and associated loss of self-esteem, the impact on activities of daily life and fear of falling. Patients may become reclusive and fearful of going outdoors and socially isolated.

■ *Increased mortality/morbidity* – An excess in mortality after vertebral fractures has been reported even in subjects who do not come to medical attention. However, the major increase in mortality occurs in symptomatic vertebral fractures. Thus in one study age adjusted relative risk of death following a vertebral fracture was 8.64 (4.45–16.74) which compared with a relative risk of 6.68 (3.08–14.52) for hip fracture.[3] Subsequent survival however declines disproportionately, probably due to the impact of coexistent comorbid conditions. The risk of reduced survival is increased following fractures due to mild or moderate trauma rather than to severe trauma. Survival after 5 years is lower for men (72%) than women (84%).

2.19 What is the impact of vertebral fracture on quality of life?

Several studies have shown the adverse effect of vertebral fractures on quality of life in terms of both psychological and physical morbidity. A recent study[22] showed that quality adjusted life years were 0.82 for 114 women with one or more vertebral fractures. The comparable value for hip fractures was 0.63. The comparator group of women without fracture had an average value of 0.91 (quality adjusted life years of 1 represents perfect health). These values were equivalent to a loss of 20 to 58 working days per year for patients with vertebral fractures. Patients reported difficulty with a large range of daily activities and had particular problems with prolonged standing, bending, transferring in and out of a car or putting socks on. The physical component of the UK's Health Status Questionnaire SF36 confirms significant impairment compared with non-fracture subjects.

Although this study did not show significant differences in the mental component scores, other studies have shown significantly increased risk of depression. An incremental impact on quality of life with a greater number of fractures is a feature of all studies for both sexes. Kanis and co-workers[21] have shown that the morbidity of patients with vertebral fractures as judged by the sickness impact profile is about one-third of that suffered by patients with hip fractures (*Fig. 2.6*).

2.20 Which types of vertebral fracture are recognised?

There are three forms of vertebral fracture: end plate, wedge and crush fracture (*Fig. 2.7*). Characteristically these occur in the mid-thoracic (maximally at T8) and thoracolumbar regions of the spine. Wedging is usually in the anterior plane.

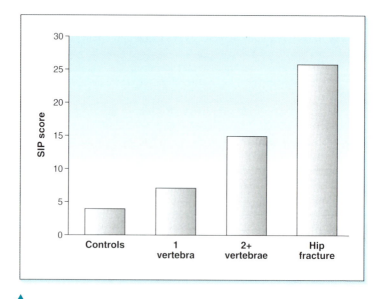

Fig. 2.6 Morbidity of patients with osteoporotic fractures assessed by the sickness impact profile (SIP). Patients with vertebral fractures had a score midway between that associated with hip fracture and that in age- and sex-matched controls. (From Kanis & McCloskey[21])

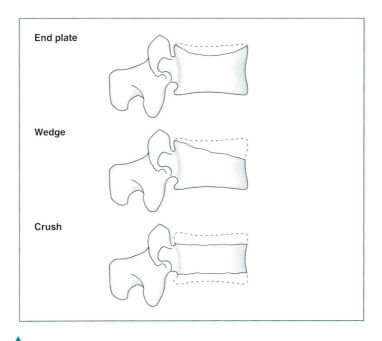

End plate

Wedge

Crush

▲

Fig. 2.7 Types of vertebral fracture.

Because of coexistent degenerative disc disease, there may be difficulties in confirming a fracture. These problems have bedevilled the study of incidence rates of fractures across different populations. Latterly it has been suggested that measurements relating to standard morphometric criteria should be used. In the clinical context, the usual rule of thumb is an 80% or less difference between the posterior and anterior vertebral heights measured on a conventional X-ray.

2.21 Which confirmatory investigations may be necessary?

Often a lateral spinal X-ray is all that is needed to confirm the diagnosis. However, in the presence of previous fractures or coexistent degenerative disc disease, a new fracture may be difficult to confirm. In this situation, isotope bone scanning or magnetic resonance images (MRI) can be useful in identifying new fractures. Thus, an isotope bone scan will show a vertebral fracture as 'hot'. The short tau inversion recovery (STIR) analysis on MRI will show vertebral oedema suggestive of recent fracture (*Fig. 2.8*). Sometimes computed tomography (CT) may be useful where there is doubt

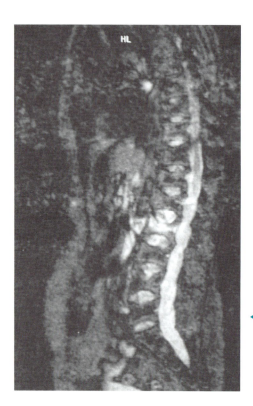

◀ **Fig. 2.8 A**, STIR sequence MRI showing collapse of all lumbar vertebrae and new fracture at L2 with marrow oedema;

A

concerning the cause of vertebral collapse and may show underlying conditions such as haemangioma or neoplasm within the vertebra.

2.22 What are the differences in vertebral fracture incidence rates between races and countries?

For the reasons already discussed, study of incidence rates of vertebral fractures between countries is difficult. Radiographic surveys suggest that between 12 and 26% of postmenopausal Caucasian women have a vertebral deformity.[23] Vertebral deformity is as frequent in Asian as in Caucasian women[24,25] but less common in Hispanics and Afro-American women. The incidence of vertebral fractures is three times that of hip fractures. However, only about a third of these come to medical attention. Overall the female to male ratio is about 2 to 1. However, the incidence of vertebral deformity in men is equal to women up until the age of 60, probably due to occupational stress and the higher risk of high trauma injuries in men. The European

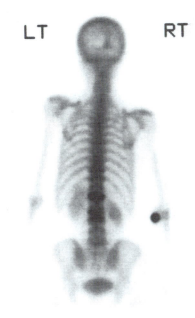

LT   RT

Fig. 2.8 Cont'd; B, isotope bone scan showing increase uptake at L1, L2 and L3.

B

Vertebral Osteoporosis Study (EVOS) of 36 countries showed an overall prevalence of morphometrically defined vertebral deformity in men and women of 12%. The prevalence increased in each sex with age, but more rapidly in women. The highest rates were found in Scandinavian countries.

Some of the variations may be attributable to physical activity and BMI differences. A strong association was found between the number of vertebral deformities and the prevalence of reported back pain and height loss.[26]

2.23 Do vertebral fractures increase the risk of subsequent fractures?

The presence of a fracture increases the risk of subsequent fracture by 4. When a fracture is clinically diagnosed, as opposed to a chance radiological finding, the risk of further vertebral fractures increases by a factor of 5.3. Even after correcting for low bone mineral density (BMD), the presence of one or more vertebral fractures increases the risk of subsequent fracture by 8.1.[27]

Overall, patients with vertebral fractures have a 20% risk of further fracture in the first year after fracture and over the next 10 years 85% are at risk. Vertebral fractures therefore warn of future vertebral fractures and also have an independent predictive power for hip fractures, i.e. the relative risk of a hip fracture increases by 3.8.

WRIST FRACTURE

2.24 How do wrist fractures occur?

Distal forearm fractures usually occur following a fall on the outstretched arm.[28] Such fractures are usually of the Colles type with displacement of the distal radial segment (*Fig. 2.9*). The pattern of incidence in women is different from vertebral or hip fractures with an increase in incidence

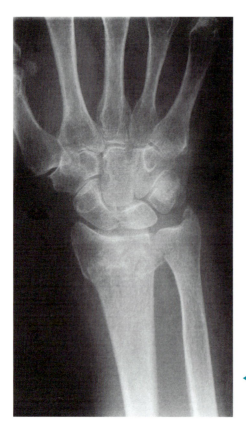

◀ **Fig. 2.9** Colles fracture with fracture of ulnar styloid.

between the ages of 40 and 65 and then subsequent stabilisation before a secondary risk in the very elderly. In men, the incidence rate is more or less constant between 20 and 80. The majority of distal forearm fractures occur in women (by a factor of 4:1).

The reason for the decline in incidence rates in later life for women is not known. It has been suggested that changes in neuromuscular coordination in women make them more liable to fall backwards in later life and thus increase the risk of hip fractures. However, this would not explain the subsequent secondary increase in such fractures in extreme old age. In the postmenopausal period, the outstretched hand is used to brace a fall.

There is a clear relationship with the seasons: typical peak incidence rates occur outdoors in cold icy conditions whereas hip fractures show less variation with the seasons and usually occur indoors.

2.25 What are the treatment options for wrist fractures?

The usual treatment is closed reduction with or without plaster immobilisation, the latter over a period of 5–6 weeks.

Where the fracture is unstable, then either external fixation or plating of the unstable section may be necessary.

It is important to restore the radial length and orientation of the distal radioulnar joint. Early mobilisation is important in reducing the risk of algodystrophy.

The early menopausal group rarely require hospitalisation. However, the likelihood of admission increases significantly with age. Thus 70% of patients with fractures of the forearm aged 85 or over require admission.

2.26 What are the consequences of wrist fractures?

Wrist fractures cause less morbidity than those of the hip or lumbar spine in the UK. They require an average three visits to hospital and costs of £494 for the acute management of the fracture have been estimated. Bony union usually occurs over 4–6 weeks.

Algodystrophy (reflex sympathetic dystrophy) is the most important complication of wrist fracture and occurs in up to 30% of cases. This usually presents with pain, stiffness and swelling of the hand with associated loss of function. Pain control is often difficult. Such patients may take many months to improve. Vigorous physiotherapy is usually advised. However, long term residual pain and stiffness may still occur. Other complications of Colles fracture are outlined in *Box 2.1*. Overall, only about 50% of patients report full functional recovery a year after wrist fracture.[29]

BOX 2.1 Complications following Colles fracture

- ■ Algodystrophy
- ■ Carpal tunnel syndrome
- ■ Malunion
- ■ Radiocarpal osteoarthritis
- ■ Deformity

2.27 What is the significance of wrist fracture in predicting further fractures?

The risk of hip fracture is increased by 1.4 in women and 2.7 in men after forearm fractures. The risk of vertebral fractures is also significantly increased – 5.2 times in women and 10.7 times in men.[30]

Thus, although after wrist fracture morbidity and functional impairment are minimal, they should act as a trigger to alert the patient and doctor to the risk of further fractures later in life. Because most wrist fractures are managed between Accident and Emergency departments and fracture clinics in hospitals and require little in the way of general practitioner input, they are often overlooked. Therefore opportunities to intervene in terms of establishing the diagnosis of osteoporosis and instituting treatment are often missed.

 PATIENT QUESTIONS

2.28 Which fractures are commonly associated with osteoporosis?

These are fractures of the wrist, spine and hip. They have the following features in common:

- ■ They are characterised by low bone density at each site and occur after relatively *trivial injury* such as a slip or stumble from a standing or sitting position.
- ■ The force needed to break the bone is often slight because of the increased fragility of bone.
- ■ Patients with osteoporosis may still have fractures after high trauma.
- ■ The pattern of fractures (i.e. their distribution in the skeleton) and the differences in fracture rates between the sexes mirrors the bone loss at these three sites, and the lower bone density in women.

Fractures may occur for reasons other than osteoporosis, such as those due to repeated stress on a bone (e.g. in athletes who overtrain) or due to weakening of the bone skeleton in association with vitamin deficiencies such

 PATIENT QUESTIONS

as vitamin D. Rarely fractures may also occur as complications of tumours or sometimes can be the presenting feature of cancer of bone or as a secondary deposit from a primary tumour elsewhere in the body. Therefore it is important that doctors consider conditions other than osteoporosis as a possible cause of fracture.

2.29 What is the distribution of osteoporotic fractures across the ages?

Characteristically the order of osteoporotic fractures in the female population is: wrist in the first two decades after the menopause; spinal fractures from the second and third decades onwards after the menopause and hip fractures in the third and fourth decades after the menopause.

In men there is no similar increase in the incidence of wrist fractures as seen in women. Wrist fractures occur throughout adult life in men and at much lower rates than for women. Spinal fractures increase at the age of about 60 and hip fractures after 70. The rate of hip fracture increases similar to that in women, but occurs about 10 years later. Overall, the number of fractures suffered by the male population is much lower than for women.

2.30 Why is there a difference in the pattern of fractures between the sexes?

The main reason for women having greater chances of fracture than men is because of their lower bone mass and because of their greater risk of falling compared to men. The cause of spinal fractures in men is thought to be at least partly occupational in origin reflecting the manual occupations of some men. There are also qualitative differences in the quality of bone between the sexes which may contribute. There are also other factors such as lower physical fitness and strength in women which may play a part in predisposition to fractures.

2.31 How do hip fractures occur?

Two factors are necessary for a fracture to occur:

1. The presence of low bone mass (osteoporosis), the causes of which are discussed in *Chapter 6*. Other major risk factors for hip fractures are shown in *Table 2.1*.
2. Sufficient force applied to bone – this usually occurs with a fall.

The risk of both osteoporosis and falling increases in the elderly. Commonly a hip fracture occurs in the home environment (rather than outside), the vast majority occurring following a fall from a standing position to one side or backwards. The fracture is a direct consequence of the force of the fall being transmitted through the bony structure of the hip. Because of the underlying weakening of the bone together with the 'unnatural' direction of the impact, the hip bone breaks more easily. The loss of bone strength and the alteration in bone structure that occurs in

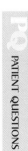

elderly women leaves them liable to such fractures. The importance of the outer 'cushion' of fat overlying the hip bone is that it provides a buffer to absorb the forces of the fall. Women of slight build, and hence with thin soft tissue around the hip, are at increased risk of fracture for this reason. Hip fractures occur at one or two sites called intracapsular or extracapsular depending on whether the fracture is within the capsule of the hip joint or not.

2.32 How are hip fractures treated?

In order to enable the patient to walk again, it is necessary to repair the bony break. This is usually done by one of two means:

1. Removal of the upper end of the thigh bone where it forms the hip joint with replacement by a new artificial joint – a hemiarthroplasty. Sometimes it is necessary to replace both the ball and the socket component of the hip by a completely new joint – an arthroplasty.
2. The fracture site may be supported by insertion of a stainless steel bar across the fracture line and held in place by screws. This is employed chiefly in the treatment of extracapsular fractures. Such fractures usually take longer to recover because the bone damage may be more extensive.

Other surgical treatments may be necessary, depending on the particular conditions that prevail, taking into account both the fitness of the patient and the nature of the fracture sustained. Whatever treatment is used, it is particularly important for the surgical procedure to be carried out as soon as possible after the fracture. Delay in surgery increases the risks of complications such as bed sores, pneumonia and blood clots (thromboses). The likelihood of a satisfactory outcome is increased if the surgery is carried out promptly and by a senior surgeon. Most operations are carried out using a general anaesthetic, but where there is particular physical frailty, an epidural (spinal) anaesthetic may be used.

2.33 What happens after a hip fracture is repaired?

After treatment it is important to get the patient moving as soon as possible since this helps both in the healing of the fracture and reducing the risk of the complications mentioned above. Patients are usually advised to use support hosiery to reduce the risk of blood clots in the legs.

Since many patients who sustain hip fractures are in the elderly, frail group, rehabilitation can be difficult and prolonged and may be carried out in a ward linked to the orthopaedic ward providing necessary rehabilitation facilities and staff – physiotherapists and occupational therapists. Initially mobility may only be possible with the help of a walking frame. The patient is encouraged to 'graduate' to walking sticks. Sometimes however, despite such care, patients do not recover their previous mobility and may lose their independence. They may require subsequent discharge to sheltered accommodation or to a nursing home.

Where patients are able to return home, it is important to identify any particular risk factors in the environment, i.e. factors which may have led to the original fall such as poor lighting or lack of grab rails, loose carpets, etc. In order to assess the home properly, an occupational therapist may visit the home prior to discharge to identify such risk factors and to enable modification of 'home hazards'.

2.34   Are there any long term issues following hip fracture?

Coexistent medical conditions which increase the risk of falls such as poor vision, parkinsonism or hypertension may also need to be addressed. Since patients who have had a hip fracture are more likely to suffer a second hip fracture, it is important to consider the use of hip protectors. Sometimes however, patients are unable to tolerate these devices. This is mainly due to discomfort, and the presence of coincident problems such as continence difficulties, poor grip, etc. Where appropriate, balance training may be given.

Advice may be directed to alter any lifestyle factors that may have contributed to the fall such as poor dietary intake of calcium and vitamin D (which is common in the elderly). Other input such as encouragement to increase exercise, desist from smoking or retard alcohol intake may reduce the risk of further fracture. Such advice and help may be given either by nursing staff, possibly a liaison fracture nurse or alternatively orthopaedic surgeon or GP.

Medical treatments such as supplemental calcium and vitamin D, bisphosphonates, hormone replacement therapy or a selective oestrogen receptor modulator (SERM) may be prescribed. Where appropriate, further investigations such as bone densitometry or allied biochemical and other tests to elucidate the cause of osteoporosis may be necessary. In general however, there is little need for confirmatory bone densitometry in the elderly group since the likelihood of osteoporosis is high.

2.35   How do spinal fractures occur?

Most spinal fractures occur 'silently', i.e. they do not cause pain and are often brought to light by chance such as an X-ray carried out because of loss of height or spinal curvature. Some patients do have low grade backache and stiffness with height loss and increased stooping of the upper back – the so called dowager's hump. However, these patients may not have osteoporosis but degenerative disc disease which in itself can give rise to spinal curvature. Loss of height is a normal consequence of ageing and is not in itself a definite sign of osteoporosis.

A minority of patients with vertebral fractures (about a third) have acute episodes of back pain usually occurring in the upper part of the spine or at the junction of the dorsal (upper) and lumbar (lower) spine. These can occur after minimal injuries such as a fall or after prolonged stooping or lifting, such as may occur after ironing or bending movements (e.g. to pick up a shopping bag). The pain can come on over a matter of a few days, but usually is dramatic, severe and sudden in onset.

Twisting or turning movements, particularly turning over in bed or sitting up, usually worsen the pain. Commonly this is felt in the central spinal area but may move or radiate to the front part of the chest or abdomen. The intensity of the pain and its association with movement has a severe restraining effect on patients' mobility, many of whom may subsequently take to their bed. Characteristically the pain after a first vertebral fracture lasts for up to 8 weeks. Unfortunately a significant proportion of patients go on to have more chronic disabling back pain. The pain is usually worse with prolonged standing, bending, stooping or lifting. The cause of the pain is complex: because of the increased stoop of the spine and the consequent extension of the head and neck, this places extra strain on the muscles of the neck and upper back which become painful. Other mechanisms include pressure on nerves which may give rise to pain around the rib cage. Those patients who have had more than one vertebral fracture have an increased risk of chronic pain after recovery from the acute pain of the fracture.

Such pain may be improved by rest and the patient may have to 'ration' periods of activity in the day with rest, usually taken on a bed or couch. In the long term, other methods to control the pain may be needed in addition to analgesics – painkillers, local physical treatments such as massage, local heat, acupuncture or the use of transcutaneous nerve stimulation (TNS) machines. Such treatment may be combined with postural exercises and techniques to lessen the stresses put on the back.

2.36 How are spinal fractures treated?

In the initial presentation, the first priority is to control the acute pain. This usually requires strong analgesics which may bring with them their own problems such as constipation, for example with codeine-containing preparations. Where the pain is very severe, additional treatment such as the use of calcitonin injections or morphine-based agents may be necessary. Some patients may require admission to hospital. However, the vast majority of patients are managed at home. Once the acute pain has been controlled, then attention shifts to the early mobilisation of patients since, as with hip fractures, prolonged immobility in this group of patients brings with it its own complications and hazards. Those who are managed in hospital may be seen and assessed by the rehabilitation team and given not only physical treatment, but advice regarding posture and exercise. Although belts have been used in the past to support the spine, their use currently is declining on the basis that they may ultimately weaken the muscles that support the spine.

In some countries a surgical procedure – vertebroplasty – may be used to improve pain. This is a technique of injecting bone cement into the vertebral fracture site through a hole drilled into the vertebra from the back, usually carried out under general anaesthetic. The validity of this procedure, i.e. its effectiveness in controlling pain, has not been extensively studied, but is increasingly used in America and Europe and may have a limited role in the treatment of pain occurring after vertebral fractures. At present, the technique is currently being evaluated in the UK, but its ultimate role in the standard treatment of vertebral fractures is not yet certain.

2.37   When and how do wrist fractures occur?

Characteristically these happen in women in the first two decades after the menopause. It is the commonest fracture up until the age of 75. They usually occur as a consequence of a fall on to the outstretched hand, usually occurring out of doors in icy conditions.

2.38   How are wrist fractures treated?

The fracture is usually of the radial bone of the forearm. The treatment consists of 'reduction', i.e. realignment of the bones, this being carried out by means of a plaster applied to the forearm and wrist after realignment of the arm under anaesthetic. However, where the bones do not readily realign then some form of 'fixation' may be needed, either in the form of a metal plate across the fracture site or rod fixed across the bones maintaining the alignment and length of the radial bone. Whatever method is used, bony healing usually occurs over about 5–6 weeks. During this time it is important to exercise the hand as much as possible in order to maintain bone strength and reduce the risk of complications.

At first there may be difficulties in performing simple tasks such as grooming and household jobs, especially if the fracture is of the dominant arm. In the elderly or frail, these problems may be very disabling. However, most patients make a good recovery. Some may suffer complications, especially the elderly. These include in particular a condition of persistent pain of the hand associated with swelling, redness of the hand and sensitivity to pain. This is called an algodystrophy. This complication is less likely when rehabilitation, in particular exercise of the hand, is carried out early and regularly after fracture.

2.39   What is the importance of a wrist fracture?

A wrist fracture may be the first indication to a patient of underlying osteoporosis. This should alert the doctor and patient to this possibility. Medical management and lifestyle changes to reduce the risk of further fractures should be considered. At this stage a bone density measurement is a useful test to confirm osteoporosis.

It is known that patients who suffer wrist fractures have a much greater risk of further fractures later in life. Thus, the confirmation of osteoporosis at the time of fracture and the use of preventative treatment may reduce the risk of future fractures. Often this 'window of opportunity' is lost since the significance of a wrist fracture may not be realised by the patient or medical staff managing the condition.

PQ PATIENT QUESTIONS

Bone physiology and pathophysiology in osteoporosis

3

3.1 How is bone formed and remodelled?

Cancellous bone is constantly being formed and replaced by two closely linked or 'coupled' processes: bone resorption and bone formation.

- *Bone resorption* – begins by the recruitment of osteoclasts to the bone surface to be resorbed. These are large multinucleate cells which are metabolically very active. They originate from haematopoietic stem cells. A resorption cavity is produced beneath each cell. The bone matrix is dissolved by the release of enzymes and acid onto the surface of bone. Once the resorption cavity has been excavated, osteoclasts then migrate away (*Fig. 3.1*).
- *Bone formation* – is carried out by osteoblasts that originate from mesenchymal stem cells which synthesise the ground substance – osteoid of bone – thus infilling the resorption cavity. Osteoid ultimately becomes mineralised under the influence of osteoblasts. Once the resorption pit has been completely filled in, osteoblasts enter a resting phase as surface cells capable of further activation as needed. Normally the amount of bone resorbed and subsequently replaced is equal in early adult life.

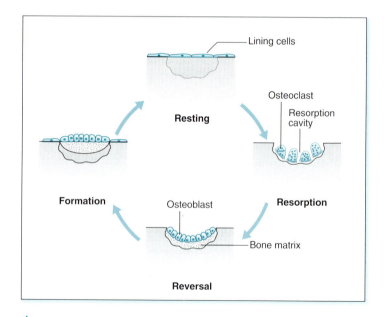

Fig. 3.1 Bone remodelling in cancellous bone.

■ In cortical bone osteoclasts arrange themselves as a cutting edge in the long axis of the bone and tunnel out a 'face' of bone which is subsequently filled in by concentric layers of osteoid secreted by osteoblasts (*Fig. 3.2*).

The remodelling cycle allows the skeleton to adjust to changes in biomechanical stresses and to repair deficits that occur in bone. Activation of a cycle normally occurs every 10 seconds in the adult skeleton. The total duration of the remodelling cycle from beginning to end is normally about 120 days.

3.2 Where does bone remodelling occur?

Both the cortical and cancellous sites of bone are actively remodelled throughout life. Since the process is surface based and because of the higher surface to volume ratio of cancellous as opposed to cortical bone (*Fig. 3.3*), the effect of remodelling is mainly evident in cancellous bone.

3.3 What changes in bone remodelling occur in osteoporosis?

In postmenopausal osteoporosis and in old age, or immobilisation, the perfect link between the amount of bone resorbed and subsequently laid

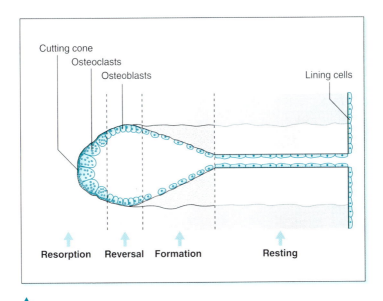

Fig. 3.2 Bone remodelling in cortical bone.

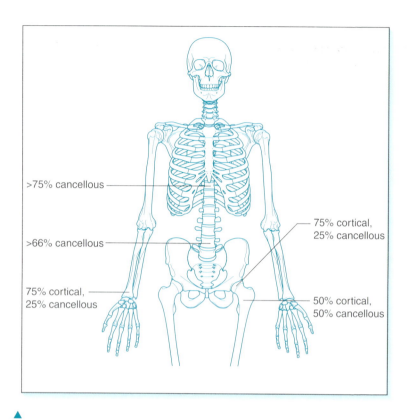

>75% cancellous

75% cortical,
25% cancellous

>66% cancellous

75% cortical,
25% cancellous

50% cortical,
50% cancellous

Fig. 3.3 Proportions of cortical and cancellous bone in the skeleton.

down is broken, with a net deficit occurring at the end of each remodelling cycle. In the postmenopausal woman, a number of factors amplify the loss of bone:

■ There is an increase in the activation frequency, i.e. the rate at which new cycles of bone resorption and subsequent bone in-filling occur. Due to the reduction of oestrogen levels amongst other factors, the net imbalance between resorption and activation combined with increased bone turnover causes an acceleration in the rate of bone loss immediately after the menopause and for several years thereafter.

■ The number of osteoclasts increases by two- to threefold at the menopause. The increased number of resorption sites means that more bone is resorbed and the pits excavated are deeper.

■ Although osteoblastic numbers also increase, their function is reduced compared to osteoclastic function and there is a relative reduction in bone deposition.

3.4 What are the structural changes that occur to bone in postmenopausal osteoporosis?

> In postmenopausal osteoporosis there is a marked reduction in trabecular numbers by up to 45%. The loss of trabeculae occurs as a result of the increased depth of the resorption cavities which ultimately weakens them and results in microfractures. The remaining trabeculae hypertrophy (*see Box 3.1*). The loss of integrity of transected trabeculae is then followed by resorption of the remnants of the unconnected struts.

In cortical bone, age-related deposition of bone at the external surface (apposition) continues to occur, but does not outweigh the effect of endosteal resorption. The result is that the external cortical 'envelope' increases, but the overall thickness of the cortex reduces.

In corticosteroid-induced osteoporosis, the structural changes that occur are different from those of postmenopausal osteoporosis. There is relative retention of the cancellous structure, but with associated marked thinning of individual trabeculae. The changes in microarchitecture of bone in male osteoporosis are also distinct from those of postmenopausal osteoporosis.

BOX 3.1 Changes in bone in postmenopausal osteoporosis

■ Increased activation frequency
■ Two- to threefold increase in osteoclasts
■ Increased depth of resorption cavities
■ Incomplete in-filling of resorption cavities
■ Trabecula plate perforation
■ Reduction in trabecular numbers
■ Hypertrophy of remaining trabeculae
■ Microfractures
■ Reduction in cortical bone thickness → loss of biomechanical strength → fracture

3.5 What is the normal pattern of bone accretion and loss during life?

Skeletal growth and mineralisation occurs throughout the first three decades of life (*see Fig. 3.4*), beginning in the foetus and affected by intrauterine influences.

■ *Phase 1* – The trajectory of skeletal growth is established during intrauterine life and the first 2 years of postnatal life.[1] These factors may have an important effect on gene expression and influence the attainment of peak bone mass, the rate of bone loss and hence risk of osteoporosis and fracture in later life. The influence of programming (a term used for the changes in structure and function caused by environmental stimuli during early development) has been the subject of recent scientific interest, with attention focused chiefly on the influence of endocrine factors including growth hormone, insulin like growth factor 1 (IGF-1), the hypothalamic–pituitary–adrenal axis and the parathyroid hormone–vitamin D axis.

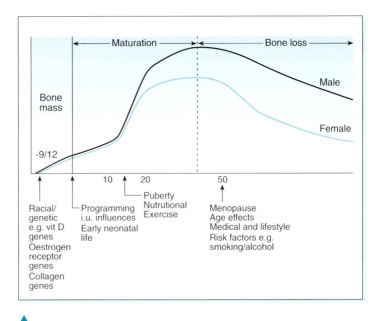

▲

Fig. 3.4 Bone mass profile throughout life (i.u., intrauterine).

■ *Phase 2* – The second major influence on bone accretion is the effect of puberty. This is accompanied by a large increase in bone mass in both sexes with girls showing an earlier increase in bone mass compared to boys. Lifestyle factors including diet and exercise have an impact on the attainment of bone density at puberty.

■ *Phase 3* – In the third phase, after completion of peak longitudinal skeletal growth, there is a period of consolidation during which peak bone mass is attained. This is achieved in the third decade of life. At this stage, peak bone mass for men is 10–15% greater than in women, depending on the site measured.

■ *Phase 4* – In the final phase, which occurs in the ageing skeleton, women have an accelerated rate of bone loss following the menopause, after which an age-related loss of bone occurs in the last few decades of life. This phase occurs in both sexes. In this stage of life the rate of bone activation is slower for both men and women compared with early adult life. In extreme old age, rates of bone loss can exceed rates of loss in the perimenopausal period.

3.6 What are the determinants of peak bone mass?

■ *Genetic and racial influences* – Studies of bone mineral content in different races, twin studies and family studies have all indicated strong genetic influences on peak bone mass.[2,3] Thus bone density in Afro-Caribbeans is greater than in Caucasians, even after adjustment for body mass index (BMI).[4] This is reflected by reduced rates of osteoporotic fractures in such groups. However, differences in osteoporotic fracture rates may also reflect differences in bone geometry between races, thus the shorter femoral neck in Afro-Caribbean subjects compared to Caucasians and Asians is associated per se with reduced fracture likelihood.[5] Other influences, particularly the different risk of falls may also account for some of the differences. Twin studies of bone mass have shown better conformity between monozygotic compared to dizygotic twins. Family studies also show a strong relationship between bone mass of mothers and their daughters. There is a strong link between maternal history of hip fracture and risk of similar fracture in daughters.[6] However, the nature of the underlying mechanism cannot be explained on the basis of bone density alone. Overall, the genetic component accounts for about 50% of bone mass. At the gene level the heritability of bone density is known to be linked to vitamin D, oestrogen receptors and collagen genes.

■ *Hormonal influences* – Sex hormones have a profound effect on the attainment of adolescent bone mass as well as strongly influencing overall skeletal size. Delayed puberty in either sex is associated with lower bone mass. In adulthood, amenorrhoea is associated with risk of osteoporosis. The impact of other hormonal influences such as oral contraceptives, breast feeding and parity remains uncertain.

■ *Nutritional factors* – The role of calcium in the attainment of peak bone mass is still a source of uncertainty and dispute. This is manifest by varying national guidelines for minimal dietary requirements for calcium. Manifestly calcium is needed for the full mineralisation of the skeleton. Deficiency of calcium and vitamin D in childhood however is associated not with osteoporosis, but osteomalacia. Calcium supplementation in puberty certainly gives rise to significant increases in bone density which may be carried into early adulthood.[7–10] The form of supplementation (e.g. as a mineral supplement, or as a calcium-rich food such as milk) may also have a bearing on the response. Other nutritional factors which impact on the attainment of peak bone mass include the energy content of food which is governed by the exercise taken by the individual. Habitual high exercise is also associated with increased bone mass.

■ *Physical activity* – As mentioned above, this plays a significant role in the attainment of peak bone mass, not only in childhood, but may be important in reducing the rate of bone loss in later life.[11,12] In adulthood, the risk of osteoporotic fractures is increased in those who exercise least. The nature of the exercise taken is important in determining the effect on bone mass: for example, weight bearing exercises is most effective, whereas swimming has no effect on bone mass. Exercise to limbs such as taken by particular sportsmen and women results in local increase in bone density and bone strength. Studies of the relationship between peak bone mass and exercise have shown that the reported levels of physical exercise in childhood impact on peak bone mass attainment. Excessive exercise in certain groups of sportswomen is associated with increased risk of osteoporosis due to secondary amenorrhoea. In this particular group the most important influence on bone mass, and liability to fracture, is not exercise, but low oestrogen or the effect of low BMI which most such women have.

3.7 What other determinants of fractures are important?

The average bone density of patients who have had fractures 'overlaps' with that of the general population. This implies that bone density is not the sole determinant of fracture (*see Box 3.2*). Factors not related to skeletal integrity – notably the risk of falling – predispose to fracture. Such factors may not be easy to assess but nonetheless, may be of particular importance in some groups of patients.

BOX 3.2 Determinants of bone strength

- Bone mineral density*
- Bone structure:
  — size
  — shape
  — geometry
  — microarchitecture
  — bone mineralisation
- Bone turnover

*BMD accounts for 75–90% of bone strength

Prior fracture per se is an independent risk factor for further fractures – independent that is, of bone density itself. This implies that qualitative differences in bone are of importance. The changes in microarchitecture that occur in postmenopausal osteoporosis include a large reduction in the number of trabeculae with hypertrophy of remaining trabeculae and loss of the cross struts. At a different level macroarchitectural influences (e.g. hip axis length) are independent predictors of risk of hip fracture. Variations in such factors may go some way to explain certain differences in incidence rates of hip fractures between populations. In particular they probably explain the higher rate of hip fracture in Scandinavian compared to Mediterranean populations.

Other quantitative influences on bone, particularly the degree of mineralisation, may have influences on fracture rates – notably in the elderly where subclinical osteomalacia may be present. Bone turnover itself is also an independent determinant of hip fracture as shown in the EPIDOS study,[13] those with the highest bone resorption markers having the greatest fracture risk. The evidence in the elderly is that bone formation is variable whereas increased bone resorption is consistently found – this uncoupling of formation and resorption may lead to microarchitectural changes that increase the risk of fracture.

3.8 What are the potential causes of osteoporosis?

Table 3.1 lists the commonest causes of osteoporosis. Conditions such as anorexia or exercise induced amenorrhoea are associated with osteoporosis due to mixed endocrine and nutritional mechanisms. Additionally there are particular groups (e.g. juveniles, patients with pregnancy-associated osteoporosis, and men) in whom the aetiology of the osteoporosis may be due to a combination of factors.

TABLE 3.1 Potential causes of osteoporosis	
Category	**Cause of osteoporosis**
Endocrine	Female hypogonadism: menopause, surgery, irradiation, hypogonadotrophism
	Men: testicular failure, hypogonadotrophism
	Thyrotoxicosis
	Excess thyroid supplementation
	Hyperparathyroidism (primary, secondary, tertiary)
	Growth hormone deficiency
	Cushing's syndrome
	Hyperprolactinaemia
	Corticosteroid treatment – oral or inhaled
General medical conditions	Chronic renal failure
	Renal osteodystrophy
	Liver failure
	Inflammatory bowel disorders
	Malabsorption disorders
	Coeliac disease
	Crohn's disease
	Rheumatoid arthritis
	Post-gastrectomy
	Malignancies, e.g. myeloma, leukaemia, lymphoma, mastocytosis
Drugs	Heparin
	Alcohol
	Cytotoxic agents
Immobility/spinal cord injury	Paraplegia
Other	Family history of hip fracture
	Genetic osteoporosis
	Smoking
	Age

3.9 What are the chief influences on the development of osteoporosis in the elderly?

Since the main impact of osteoporosis is seen in the elderly, the important influences in determining susceptibility to osteoporosis and fracture (*see Box 3.3*) have been closely examined:

■ *Changes in bone turnover* – Over their lifespan, women lose about 42% of spinal bone mass and 58% of hip bone mass.[14] Bone turnover in the

---

BOX 3.3 Factors contributing to osteoporosis of the elderly

- Nutritional, e.g.
  - — malnutrition
  - — low vitamin D or calcium in diet
  - — intestinal resistance to vitamin D
  - — impaired hydroxylation of 25 (OH) vitamin D
  - — reduced absorption of calcium from the gut
  - — reduced production of vitamin D in skin
- Hormonal, e.g.
  - — decline in oestrogen
  - — decline in testosterone
  - — reduction in growth hormone secretion
  - — secondary hyperparathyroidism
  - — reduction in adrenal androgen
- Chronic conditions associated with osteoporosis, e.g.
  - — rheumatoid arthritis
  - — chronic renal failure
  - — liver disease
  - — myeloma
  - — hyperthyroidism
  - — malabsorption
- Medication, e.g.
  - — steroid use
  - — anticonvulsants
  - — use of anti-gonadotrophin drugs
  - — thyroxine
- Lifestyle factors, e.g.
  - — smoking
  - — excess alcohol
  - — immobility

---

very old is significantly higher than in the postmenopausal group.[15] Those with the highest bone resorption markers have the greatest risk of fracture, independent of bone mass. As discussed, bone formation markers show no consistent changes in the elderly, i.e. the link between formation and resorption in the elderly is uncoupled.

- *Nutritional* – Low calcium intake in the elderly gives rise to secondary hyperparathyroidism with resultant mobilisation of calcium from the skeleton. This is compounded by reduced intake of vitamin D which is common in the old. Skin conversion of endogenous vitamin D to its active metabolites is reduced. Also there is less renal conversion of 25 hydroxyvitamin D to 1,25 dihydroxyvitamin D. These changes in vitamin D metabolism lead to a net reduction in calcium absorption from the gut. Such abnormalities in calcium and vitamin D metabolism in the elderly can be corrected by supplemental vitamin D and calcium. Additionally, malnutrition – including vitamin K deficiency – can lead to acceleration of bone resorption.
- *Hormonal* – There are significant relationships between bone mineral density (BMD) in elderly men and women with oestrogen and

androgen levels.[16] In men the association between oestradiol and BMD is stronger than with testosterone and BMD.[17] Age-related reduction in both oestrogen and androgen contribute to the decline in BMD in both sexes. Other adverse influences on bone formation in the elderly skeleton include changes in the growth hormone/IGF axis and reduced adrenal androgen production.

■ *Other influences* – Lifestyle factors such as smoking and alcohol intake also contribute to the risk of osteoporosis in the elderly.

Although bone density is obviously important in the elderly in determining the risk of fracture, other influences, notably the liability to falls, are more important relative to bone density in determining fracture risk.

3.10 How do smoking and alcohol affect bone mass?

Alcohol in excess appears to be a risk factor for osteoporosis, particularly in men. This may be mediated by a direct toxic effect on osteoblasts with consequent reduced bone formation. Other contributing factors are likely to be the associated nutritional deficiencies seen in alcoholics including a low vitamin D and protein intake. Reduced free testosterone may also be important. The classical presentation of osteoporosis in alcoholics is as rib fractures on chest X-ray. Acute alcohol toxicity is followed by hypoparathyroidism with hypercalcuria. Subsequent 'rebound' hyperparathyroidism may lead to further loss of bone.

There has been no evidence to suggest that *moderate* intake of alcohol is detrimental to bone or increases risk of fracture. In fact, such intake may be protective against bone loss at the hip and may reduce the risk of vertebral fracture.

Smoking increases the risk of osteoporotic fractures in both men and women.[18] The effect may be partly mediated by a reduction in BMI with associated reduction in soft tissue over the trochanter. Reduced bone formation and increased resorption are likely to be due to decreased oestrogen production compounded by increased oestrogen degradation.[19] Female smokers have an earlier menopause which per se is associated with increased risk of osteoporosis.

3.11 How does oestrogen reduction at the menopause induce changes in bone remodelling?

Female sex hormones have a profound effect, not only in the attainment of peak bone mass in men and women, but in the maintenance of bone density. The importance of female sex hormones is seen in conditions where reduced levels occur, for example in anorexia-induced amenorrhoea or the effects of gonadotrophin inhibitors which are associated with low bone mass.

Oestrogen deficit after the menopause appears to be the main cause of osteoporosis and is also important in the aetiology of osteoporosis in men. The uncoupling of resorption and formation of bone after the menopause may be mediated by the promotion of cytokines in the bone marrow. Falls in oestrogen are associated with increases in tumour necrosis factor alpha (TNFα) and interleukins 1 and 6 (IL1 and IL6).[20,21] Oestrogen has an inhibitory effect on osteoclastic function such that reduction in oestrogen increases osteoclastic numbers and their resorptive activity.

 PATIENT QUESTIONS

3.12 How is bone formed?

Bone is made up of a hard outer 'skin' of cortical bone within which is a lighter structure resembling the struts of a bridge – cancellous bone. Between these struts lies the bone marrow. Bone is formed initially in the foetus and continues to be laid down in childhood with significant increases in the size and density of bone occurring during puberty. Bone growth occurs both in length and in circumference. Hormonal changes during adolescence cause bones to accelerate growth in length with a consequent growth 'spurt'. On completion of puberty the bones cease growing and the overall skeletal size is then fixed.

The production of bone is under the influence of two types of bone cell which work in close collaboration with each other in a cyclical way: bone resorbing cells or osteoclasts act to excavate bone pits in the first step of the remodelling process; bone forming cells or osteoblasts repair the deficit in the bone produced by osteoclasts. The 'purpose' of this process is to enable bone to adapt to the varying stresses and strains put on it during life. During childhood, the balance between bone formation and bone resorption is in favour of the former. This process is increased further during puberty resulting in big gains in bone mass at this time. The increase in bone mineral content results in increased bone strength. Bone therefore is not inert, but a living structure which throughout life adapts to the mechanical stresses put on it.

3.13 What are the changes that occur to bone in osteoporosis?

In postmenopausal women, bone is lost from the skeleton. This occurs because of a disturbance in the usual balance between bone formation and bone loss. Thus, after the end of each 'cycle', instead of the excavated pit of bone being completely filled in, there is a deficit. Ultimately this culminates in an overall loss of bone. Additionally the structure of the remaining bone is defective, mainly due to loss of the cancellous component of bone with resultant increased liability to fracture. Because the maximal loss of bone in menopausal women occurs at the cancellous site, structures rich in such bone (e.g. the vertebrae) become more susceptible to fracture. This accounts for the increased incidence of vertebral fractures in the second decade after the menopause. Loss of cortical bone is more belated and this is ultimately associated with increased risk of fracture at cortical rich sites such as the hip. Characteristically, the rate of hip fractures increases in the seventh and eighth decades of life.

3.14 What is peak bone mass and why is it important?

The maximum amount of bone in the skeleton is achieved in the third decade of life. The amount and strength of bone has a direct bearing on the likelihood of fractures. The higher the peak bone density in adult life therefore, the less likelihood of fractures in later life. After middle age, both men and women lose bone, women particularly so after the menopause. Since peak bone mass in women is lower than in men, the risk of fracture is already greater in women than in men prior to the effect of the menopause.

Men have larger and denser bones and although bone density declines in men, there is no equivalent sudden decline as there is for women. The decline in bone density in men is slow and gradual over many years.

3.15 What are the osteoporosis-related fractures?

The common sites for fractures to occur are the wrist, the spine and the hip (*see Ch. 2*).

3.16 Are genetic factors important in determining peak bone mass?

The main determinants of bone mass are genetic. However, influences on the growing baby in the womb as well as in the first 2 years of life are important in determining bone mass. Overall the genetic component of peak bone mass accounts for about 50% of total bone mass. The remainder is determined by the influences of hormones and nutritional and physical factors such as the amount of exercise taken, the amount of calcium in the diet, etc.

3.17 What is the normal bone mass profile throughout life?

■ Bone is first formed in the foetus within the mother's womb. As mentioned, the potential amount of bone and to some extent the quality of bone of an individual is set by genetic influences inherited from each parent. Thus, the risk of developing osteoporosis and associated fracture is to some degree predetermined.

■ The *actual* amount of bone deposited in early life, particularly the first 2 years after birth, is influenced by environmental effects within the womb. Factors which induce stress in the developing foetus have a profound effect on bone development. The mechanism by which bone is influenced by such factors is called 'programming'. The same mechanism predisposes to the development of other chronic disorders in later life such as coronary artery disease, diabetes and high blood pressure. During development within the womb, the influence of nutrition – in particular adequate protein, carbohydrate and mineral intake – is important in determining optimal bone formation. The impact of programming on the attainment of peak bone mass in adults has been studied by using the birth weight which reflects the combined effects of programming, genetic and nutritional factors. This shows that there is a relationship between low birth weight and reduced bone density in young adults.

■ The second big influence on bone growth in early life is the effect of puberty. This usually begins for girls at about the age of 13 and in boys a year later. The development of the skeleton in children is strongly influenced by the sex hormones, oestrogen and testosterone, both of which increase the net gain of bone in each bone cycle. During puberty, these cause an increase in the rate of bone size and ultimately the amount of bone mineral in the bony 'envelope'. Once puberty is completed, the continuing effects of the sex hormones on the skeleton lead to a gradual increase in bone mass due to further calcium deposition in bone. This continues up until bone mass is achieved in the third decade of life. Delayed onset of puberty, for any reason, may result in lower bone mass in late childhood and this effect will be carried forward into adult life.

■ In early adulthood, bone mass gradually increases as indicated and reaches a peak – the *peak bone mass* – in the late twenties in each sex.

3.18   What are the causes of osteoporosis?

Much is now known about the causation of osteoporosis, so that it is possible to identify patients in danger of osteoporosis by the use of risk factors. These essentially boil down to *fixed* or unchangeable factors and others which may be altered – *changeable* factors. It is important to note that the possession of a risk factor for osteoporosis or fracture does not mean that an individual possessing such risk factor will inevitably have osteoporosis. It merely implies a greater chance of osteoporosis than those who do not have such a risk factor. Conversely, some patients with osteoporosis may have no identifiable risk factors at all. The usefulness of risk factors to doctors is that it enables them to identify patients at potential risk, i.e. to select patients for bone density measurements and so to help direct treatment where it is most needed.

3.19   What are the risk factors for osteoporosis?

There are two types of risk factor in osteoporosis: fixed and changeable.

Fixed risk factors

■ *Sex* – Women are more prone to osteoporosis than men. In general, bone density in women falls after the menopause, although there are variations in peak bone density and the rate of bone loss between women. Nevertheless, overall there is an increased risk of osteoporosis after the menopause. This together with the fact that increasing numbers of women reach old age and also 'accumulate' other independent risk factors for osteoporosis, means that the brunt of the condition is borne by women in later life.

■ *Genetic factors* – The influence of genetic factors is manifest by increased risk of vertebral or hip fractures in the daughters of women who have had such fractures. On the one hand this could be seen as a rather negative association. On the other hand, knowing that there is an increased risk of fracture in such patients gives them and their doctor an advantage in enabling preventative strategies to be put in place, for example modification of lifestyle factors, the use of drugs, the reduction in risk of falling, etc., all of which may contribute to lowering the risk of fracture. The impact of genetic factors is also seen in the different risks of osteoporosis seen in different races such as the reduced risk seen in those of African origin compared with the rates in Caucasians, Asians and Chinese. Overall, the rate of hip fracture in Caucasian women is twice that of African women.

■ *Age* – After peak bone density is reached in early adulthood, a decline in bone density occurs in both sexes.

■ *Body size* – Small, thin men and women are at an increased risk of osteoporosis and fracture than taller, heavier people. Body size is governed to a large degree by genetic factors, chiefly the influence of parental height, but is also affected by influences on growth within the womb and nutrition in childhood.

Changeable risk factors

■ *Hormonal factors* – In women bone density and hence bone strength are linked to the total exposure bone has had to the female hormone oestrogen. Factors which either delay the onset of normal puberty or cause an early menopause increase the risk of osteoporosis. Therefore, delayed onset of, or irregular or infrequent periods, or cessation of periods for longer than 6 months, and early menopause, are all risk factors for osteoporosis. Whatever the cause of low oestrogen, it is usually possible to counteract the deficit either by replacement with hormonal treatments or related drugs or by using alternative agents which can either maintain or improve bone stock (e.g. bisphosphonates).

In men, reduction of the circulating male hormone testosterone can be associated with low bone density. Just as in women, late production of testosterone results in delayed puberty. A fall in the normal circulating levels in adulthood may cause reduced bone mineral content. One of the commonest causes of low testosterone in men is alcoholism. Just as in women, the level of testosterone in the blood can be measured and it is possible to replace testosterone by tablet, injection or patch.

■ *Dietary factors* – Calcium is the chief mineral found in bone. Intuitively, one would presume that patients who have low calcium in their diet would be more at risk of osteoporosis. The evidence for such effects is not as strong as one would expect and remains a source of contention. The influences of calcium on bone strength appear to be strongest at the extremes of age, i.e. in children and the elderly. The reason for some of the controversy about the importance of calcium in the diet is partly to do with the ability of the body to adapt to low calcium in the diet by increasing absorption of what calcium there is and to reduce the amount of calcium excreted. Thus the skeleton is protected from calcium deficiency, at least to some extent. Nevertheless, it is generally agreed that calcium is an important element, particularly at times of rapid bone growth such as during pregnancy, at puberty and when breast feeding. As people become older, the efficiency of calcium absorption from the gut declines and calcium supplementation in the elderly is usually advised.

■ *Vitamin D* – Absorption of calcium from the gut and its excretion in the urine is heavily influenced by vitamin D. In the body this is produced by the effects of ultraviolet light on the skin. About 15–20 minutes of exposure of the face and arms to sunlight per day during the summer months should be sufficient to 'stock up' on vitamin D for the year. Since elderly people are often unable to get outside and, coincidentally may not be taking a diet adequate in vitamin D, they are more prone to low vitamin D levels. In this situation, the response of the body is to maintain the calcium level in the blood by removing calcium from bone and hence osteoporosis may occur. Supplementation of the diet with vitamin D together with calcium in the elderly may therefore stave off the risk of osteoporosis.

■ *Other dietary factors* – Dietary factors which may be of importance in influencing the risk of osteoporosis include: protein – needed for tissue growth and repair; carbohydrate – needed for energy; and vitamin C – again needed for wound repair.

■ *Physical activity* – For bone to attain and maintain its maximal strength, it requires stresses and strains to be put on it – such as occur in everyday activities and with exercise. Those who are immobile or unable to exercise (e.g. with a paralysis or an illness causing the patient to be bed ridden) can become osteoporotic. The strains on bone are applied by muscle action or gravity. The effects of gravity can be maximised by weight bearing exercises such as jogging or running. It is important that exercise is weight bearing since if it is not, the effect on bone strength may be slight even though muscular strength may improve. Swimming does not increase bone strength. Exercise is also important in reducing the risk of fracture since increased physical fitness reduces the risk of falling. Advice about the type and duration of exercise to be taken should be sought from a physiotherapist or doctor knowledgeable in this area.

3.20   What other lifestyle factors can increase the risk of fracture?

■ *Smoking* – Smoking appears to increase the risk of fractures in both men and women. In women the effect may be due to reduced oestrogen levels. Women who smoke are likely to have an earlier menopause than those who do not, thus the risk of bone loss at an earlier age than usual is

PQ PATIENT QUESTIONS

increased (in the UK the average age of the menopause is 50). The increased risk of fractures in smokers may be partly related to the fact that smokers in general are thinner than non-smokers and may carry less fat to protect the hip from the trauma of a fall.

■ *Alcohol excess* – Excessive intake of alcohol is associated with osteoporosis. Doctors may first be aware of alcohol excess by the chance finding of rib fractures on a chest X-ray. Whilst it is clear that taken in excess, alcohol is associated with an increased risk of osteoporosis and fractures, in smaller doses there may be a protective effect on bone density, particularly if alcohol is taken in the form of red wine.

3.21 What are the chief factors which increase the risk of osteoporosis in the elderly?

The main categories which increase the risk of osteoporosis in the elderly are shown in *Box 3.3*. It can be seen that there are a number of factors which give rise to increased risk of osteoporosis, some of which are interlinked. It is often the case that patients who present with a fracture have several factors which in combination have contributed to low bone density and fracture. An example is an old person from a nursing home who has age-related bone loss, who has a reduced intake of calcium and vitamin D, who may be immobile because of arthritis and who has other factors which increase the likelihood of falls (e.g. poor eyesight or dizziness).

How to detect and diagnose osteoporosis

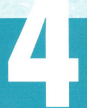

4

4.1 Which preventative strategies could be used to reduce fractures?

Since osteoporosis is widely prevalent in the population, two possible preventative strategies have been considered:

1. A population-based approach by which risk factors in the general population are identified and modified, bone mineral density (BMD) being such a risk factor. It has been shown that if the BMD of the general population were increased by 10% this would reduce the risk of fractures by 50%.[1]

2. A case finding strategy by which particular subjects possessing risk factors are identified and treated followed by drug intervention or lifestyle modification or both. Those with low BMD or propensity to fall, or with particular medical conditions associated with osteoporosis would be identified and targeted for interventions aimed at reducing the risk of fracture.

These two approaches are not mutually exclusive. At present however, for a variety of reasons shown in *Box 4.1*, the population-based approach is not favoured. The case finding approach is promoted by the World Health Organization (WHO), the International Osteoporosis Foundation and the American Society for Bone and Mineral Research as well as UK groups (*see Appendix 1*). The detection of osteoporosis does require an integrated approach between primary and secondary care, including social services.

4.2 Who is at risk of osteoporosis?

The major risk factors for osteoporosis are indicated in *Table 3.1* (p. 52). These were drawn from consensus opinion. In addition to these, lifestyle

---

BOX 4.1 Problems with population-based prevention

■ Strength of association of risk factors with osteoporosis is variable
■ Ability to influence population lifestyle (and hence risk factors) is limited and compliance with lifestyle modification is variable
■ The duration and impact of some lifestyle modifications on fracture prevention is disputed (e.g. exercise)
■ The impact of a population-based approach to modification of lifestyle has not been formally evaluated
■ The impact of interventions may be maximal only in those at the extremes of risk
■ Some risk factors are not modifiable (e.g. hip geometry, body size, ethnicity, etc.)

risk factors may be important, including smoking, alcohol intake, and the other factors shown in *Table 3.1*. Patients in these groups are at increased risk of *low bone density* and *fracture*. The Royal College of Physicians (RCP) report of 1999[2] suggested that these should be used to identify patients at risk to confirm or refute the diagnosis of osteoporosis by bone densitometry.

It is important to realise that risk factors per se do not mean that osteoporosis is inevitable in an individual. The evidence for risk factors is based on studies of populations. These have shown that the use of risk factors alone, or in combination, do not provide sufficient sensitivity or specificity to reliably categorise patients. The RCP recommendations suggest that the presence of a fragility fracture – defined as a fracture from standing height, and including a prevalent vertebral deformity – are strong, independent risk factors which merit treatment independent of BMD assessment. Such risk factors are *non-specific* in the sense of categorising potential groups of patients at risk of low BMD and general risk of fracture. There are however, *specific* risk factors for particular fractures (e.g. those derived from the Study of Osteoporotic Fractures[3] which apply to the hip). Risk factors for falls are of chief relevance in the elderly.

4.3   Which particular groups are at greatest risk of osteoporosis and fractures?

Age alone has a profound effect on the risk of fracture independent of its association with decreasing BMD. A 10 year increase in age is associated with a 94% increase in fracture risk compared to which a drop in BMD of 0.1 g/cm^2 is equivalent to a 44% increased risk of fracture.[4] BMD is less important in determining the risk of fracture in the elderly than the risk of falling.

Residents of nursing homes are at highest risk of osteoporosis since they are usually frail and elderly, and have multiple risk factors. In practice, the maximum risk of fracture (usually a hip fracture) is within the first few months of a patient taking up residency. This reflects the difficulties elderly patients have in accommodating to new surroundings. The admission of patients to nursing homes therefore presents opportunities to identify those at risk of osteoporosis and fracture. Standards for residential and nursing homes for elderly people require an assessment of health and personal care. These should include an assessment of the risk of falling.

Although evidence of the cost effectiveness of applying fall reduction strategies in the community is lacking, in the nursing home environment it is prudent to identify those at risk followed by interventions to reduce the risk of falls or to lessen the effect of the fall by the use of hip protectors.

4.4 What is the role of risk factors other than BMD in the assessment of fracture risk?

BMD is an important and measurable risk factor for fractures. However, other risk factors are also important. Those for hip fracture are listed in *Table 2.3* (p. 25) and are taken from the Study of Osteoporotic Fractures (SOF)[3] which is an important landmark study. Independent risk factors for hip fractures were deduced from this study. These showed amongst others, that women who used anticonvulsant drugs were at highest risk; a maternal history of hip fracture was also an independent risk factor.

Other risk factors are related to physical fitness: on feet for ≤ 4 hours per day, inability to get up from a chair without use of arms, and resting pulse of > 80/min. When the impact of individual risk factors was studied, it appeared that these factors had only a moderate impact on the risk of fracture. However, when combined with a measurement of bone density (in this case the os calcis) then the risk of fracture increased significantly. Thus, the rate of hip fractures per 1000 woman years increased to 27.3 for women with more than five risk factors who had the lowest BMD results compared to 1.1 with the highest BMD and up to two risk factors.[3]

Subsequent reanalysis of the data from the SOF shows that the long list of risk factors can be condensed to a more manageable number, these being: smoker, low body weight, previous fragility fracture and maternal history of hip fracture.

The use of risk factors, either alone or in combination, shows relatively weak specificity and sensitivity, i.e. they are poor at indicating either low bone mineral density or risk of fracture. Common, but weak risk factors such as smoking have a greater influence on risk scores than stronger, but less common risk factors such as steroid use or hypogonadism.

The usefulness of risk factors varies according to age group, for example those for falls (e.g. poor vision, reduced mobility, use of sedatives) are stronger predictors of fracture in the elderly than in younger subjects.[5]

4.5 How to detect those at risk of osteoporosis

Patients presenting with the ultimate expression of osteoporosis – i.e. fractures – are usually managed in secondary care (with the exception of vertebral fractures, the majority of which do not come to clinical attention). Asymptomatic osteoporosis may be present for several decades before a fracture occurs. This presents an opportunity to implement detection and preventative strategies in primary care to reduce the incidence of fractures.

Since risk factors for osteoporosis are well established, it is possible to put in place systems to identify those at risk. Ideally a collaborative approach can be used to identify and manage such people. Opportunities for patient identification include the following:

- *New patient questionnaires* – Patients joining a practice provide an opportunity to identify those with risk factors for osteoporosis.
- *Review of hospital letters* – This provides an opportunity to highlight those with fractures or with medical conditions associated with osteoporosis.
- *Review of repeat prescriptions* – This will identify patients receiving corticosteroids or other relevant medications, for example HRT or those receiving treatments which induce hypogonadism (e.g. the management of prostate cancer). Patients thus identified as being at risk may have their case notes reviewed and the patient formally assessed either by a practice nurse or primary care physician/general practitioner (GP). This approach cannot identify all such patients already in the practice unless it is possible to carry out a review of case notes. Computer-based auditing systems may make it possible to identify such patients at risk from practice records.
- *Nursing homes* – It may not be possible to identify patients in nursing homes where the risk of osteoporosis is particularly high, but where contact with GPs may be low. In this setting, as discussed (*see Q. 11.10*), assessment of risk of fracture should be undertaken at the time of transfer or admission.
- *Well Woman Clinics* – These clinics offer an opportunity to assess osteoporosis risk. Management should relate not only to possible bone densitometry and drug management, but also to lifestyle changes.
- *Other opportunities* to consider the possibility of osteoporosis include serendipitous case finding in the course of consultations for unrelated conditions or during the course of health promoting activities and by audits of practice drug prescribing.

4.6   How is the diagnosis of osteoporosis established?

Since the basis of diagnosis is by the measurement of BMD by dual energy X-ray absorptiometry (DXA), referral for measurement is usually necessary. Other techniques such as computed tomography, ultrasound and peripheral DXA (pDXA) should be used only where DXA is not available. Obviously the ability to confirm the diagnosis of osteoporosis will depend on access to such equipment which, even now in the UK, is limited in certain parts of the country.

To a certain extent, the age of the patient is also a determining factor in the use of DXA. In the early postmenopausal group BMD measurement at spine, hip or forearm is of use in determining overall fracture risk. In the elderly group, where the most important fracture is that of the hip, measurement at this site is most relevant. BMD or ultrasonic measurements at the os calcis are also useful predictors of hip fracture.

4.7   What other investigations should be undertaken?

Once the diagnosis is established, it is necessary for a clinician to review the patient (*see Box 4.2*). A general medical examination is usually necessary and a history should be taken to determine conditions associated with osteoporosis. It is important to identify other factors which may increase the risk of fracture, notably the risk of falling. Medical examination should include a record of height and the presence of kyphosis. Physical examination should also focus on risk factors for falls including evidence of muscle wasting and weakness, postural instability or poor coordination and visual deficit. Simple testing of muscular strength should include testing the

---

BOX 4.2 Evaluation of patients at risk of osteoporosis

- Demographics:
  - age
  - sex
  - ethnicity
  - body mass index
- History:
  - early menopause
  - low trauma fracture
  - back pain
  - height loss
  - kyphosis
  - anorexia
  - secondary causes of osteoporosis
- Other risk factors:
  - smoker
  - alcohol excess
  - low calcium intake
  - low levels of exercise
  - history of falls
- Family history:
  - hip or vertebral fractures
- Physical examination:
  - general – measurement of height
  - presence of kyphosis/scoliosis
  - postural hypotension

- mental status evaluation – presence of dementia, depression
- visual assessment – glaucoma, cataract, macular degeneration
- cardiac evaluation – arrhythmia, valvular disorders, bruits
- neurological examination – focal deficit, CVA, neuropathy, tremor, increased body sway
- musculoskeletal evaluation – arthritis, muscle wasting or weakness, inability to get up from a chair without using the arms
- foot abnormalities – foot deformities, unsafe footwear
- Investigations:
  - low bone mineral density
  - abnormal ultrasound measurement
  - osteopenic X-ray
  - presence of vertebral fracture on X-ray

ability to get up from a chair without the use of arms (associated with increased risk of hip fracture). Body sway is also a predictor of fracture independent of BMD.

Underlying causes of osteoporosis are more commonly found in men than in women; 50% of men with vertebral fractures have an underlying cause such as hypogonadism, steroid use or alcohol excess.[6,7] The types of investigation undertaken will depend on the clinical context. Routine investigations include those listed in *Box 4.3*.

4.8 What is the role of X-rays of the spine in the evaluation of patients with osteoporosis?

X-rays of the spine may be reported as showing evidence of osteopenia in the absence of an overt vertebral fracture; however it is unwise to rely on an X-ray diagnosis of osteoporosis since the incidence of confirmed osteoporosis in patients referred with radiological osteopenia is only 50%.

The main use of spinal X-rays is in the confirmation of a vertebral fracture in patients with a dorsal kyphosis or those with height loss and back pain. X-rays may show features of osteoporosis such as accentuation of the vertical trabeculae (due to hypertrophy of the vertical, and relative loss of horizontal trabeculae) or diffuse loss of trabeculae. The interpretation of these changes is subjective and, without a concomitant vertebral fracture, cannot in themselves be used to diagnose osteoporosis. X-rays may be used after the establishment of the diagnosis of osteoporosis by DXA in the subsequent work-up of patients to assess their future

---

BOX 4.3 Investigations of patients with osteoporosis

- Full blood count
- PV, ESR
- Biochemical profile including:
  — alkaline phosphate
  — calcium
  — phosphate
  — urea and creatinine
- Thyroid function tests
- Serum and urine electrophoresis*
- 24 hour urine calcium*
- Testosterone, SHBG, FSH-LH*
- Prostate specific antigen*
- Endomysial antibodies*

*These tests are applicable depending on the clinical context.

fracture risk. The importance of prevalent vertebral fractures lies in the fact that they have a summative effect on the risk of further fracture. Vertebral fractures are important indicators of potential fractures of all sorts (*Box 4.4*).

4.9 What is the importance of defining secondary causes of osteoporosis?

Although for women the likelihood of secondary causes of osteoporosis is only about 30%, for men it is about 50%. Identification of underlying causes of osteoporosis in themselves sometimes results in an improvement in bone density and lower fracture risk after treatment of the primary condition. For example, following the detection of coeliac disease, the advent of a gluten-free diet will often lead to an increase in BMD. Similarly, correction of lifestyle factors may reduce the risk of further bone loss. The impact of changes in lifestyle factors such as increased exercise, desisting from smoking and increased calcium intake is impossible to assess on an individual basis; nevertheless, they offer an opportunity for patients to take a hand in their own management.

It is also important that consideration is given to conditions which may mimic osteoporosis (*Table 4.1*). Such conditions may present with features of bone loss and fractures.

4.10 What is the role of biochemical markers in the assessment of osteoporosis?

Such markers of bone formation or resorption have no place in the routine assessment of patients with osteoporosis. Their role is under development and review and may ultimately be helpful in the monitoring of drug effects and assessment of patients who fail to respond to treatment, or in special groups of patients. Usually such investigations are carried out at specialist centres.

BOX 4.4 Fracture risk of patients with vertebral deformities on X-ray (95% confidence intervals)

- Any fracture 2.8:
  — men 4.2 (3.2–5.3)
  — women 2.7 (2.4–3.0)
- Vertebral fracture 12.6 (11–14)
- Hip fracture 2.3 (1.8–2.9)
- Wrist fracture 1.6 (1.0–2.4)

TABLE 4.1 Conditions which may mimic osteoporosis

Condition	Tests
Osteomalacia (e.g. due to impaired intake of vitamin D, impaired PO_4, renal handling, chronic anticonvulsant use)	Calcium PO_4 Vitamin D Parathyroid hormone
Myeloma	Bence Jones protein Serum electrophoresis Electrophoresis
Metastatic or primary tumours	X-ray Isotope bone scan MRI Tumour markers (e.g. prostate specific antigen)
Skeletal abnormalities (e.g. Scheuermann's disease)	X-ray

4.11 How else can care for patients with osteoporotic fractures be improved?

Evidence suggests that only a minority of patients with fractures are referred for assessment of osteoporosis. In one study from Glasgow only 14% and 6.3% of patients with hip and wrist fractures respectively had undergone DXA measurement or been offered treatment to reduce fracture risk.[8] As a result of these findings, a fracture liaison service was set up.

In this model (*Fig. 4.1*), a senior nurse, in conjunction with the physician in charge of the bone metabolism unit, is responsible for identifying patients with fracture by attending daily ward rounds with the orthopaedic consultants and their nursing staff. Fracture clinics are also reviewed. Following this, patients are counselled concerning their risk of further fracture and provided with the necessary information relating to osteoporosis and its management. Treatment protocols are applied and where necessary bone densitometry arranged.

Clinics run by the fracture liaison nurse offer interpretation of the DXA scans, consideration of other risk factors and advice about management including lifestyle modification and rehabilitation. Where necessary, other investigations are requested. Subsequent communication with a patient's GP and orthopaedic surgeon incorporates bone density results, analysis of fracture risk and treatment recommendations.

An audit of this service showed that it was appreciated by patients and GPs alike. A model service such as this goes a considerable way to covering the 'gap' between primary and secondary care. Until the service was

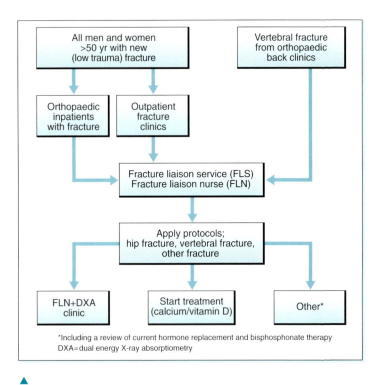

Fig. 4.1 The fracture liaison service. (From McLellan et al.[9])

introduced, those patients with a maximum risk of further fracture had not been systematically assessed or treated.[9]

4.12 What special groups of patients are there?

Special groups of patients include men, children and women with osteoporosis of pregnancy.

MEN

The largest group of patients identified at risk of osteoporosis in general practice are postmenopausal women. The BMD definitions of osteoporosis and osteopenia were established for women. Nevertheless, in practice the same criteria are used to define osteoporosis and osteopenia in men and to categorise patients' risk of fracture. Studies have shown that the prevalence of osteoporosis at the hip, spine and forearm of men over 50 is comparable to the lifetime risk of fracture at such sites. About 50% of men who present with low trauma vertebral fractures have bone density measurements in the osteoporotic range, and about 40% have osteopenia.[10,11] Treatment of osteoporosis is usually directed to men who have had low trauma fractures and evidence of osteoporosis or osteopenia. Secondary causes of osteoporosis in men (*Box 4.5*) should be considered. As for women, careful history taking and physical examination and subsequent investigations should be carried out. In addition to the usual biochemical and allied tests, a number of particular tests apply to men, for example testosterone, sex hormone binding globulin (SHBG) and prostate specific antigen (PSA). Other tests such as bone marker studies or bone biopsies may be necessary. Most men with osteoporosis should be referred to a specialist bone clinic.

CHILDREN

Osteoporosis is a rare condition in children, who usually present between 5 and 13 years of age with vertebral crush fractures. Certain inherited conditions, the commonest of which is osteogenesis imperfecta, may also present in childhood with multiple fractures, as do rarer conditions such as hypophosphatasia (*Box 4.6*).

BOX 4.5 Osteoporosis in men – possible causes

- Youth:
    - — delayed puberty
    - — genetic influences
    - — low calcium
    - — low exercise
- Middle and old age:
    - — reduction in free testosterone
    - — reduction in growth hormone/IGF-1
    - — reduced aromatisation of testosterone
    - — reduction in oestradiol
    - — reduction in adrenal androgen
    - — hyperparathyroidism
    - — reduced physical activity
    - — low calcium intake
    - — vitamin D deficiency
    - — low exercise activity
    - — smoking
    - — drug effects – steroids, gonadotrophin blockers, alcohol

---

BOX 4.6 Osteoporosis in children – possible causes

- Genetic:
  — Turner's syndrome
  — Klinefelter's syndrome
  — osteogenesis imperfecta
  — homocystinuria
  — hypophosphatasia
  — hypercalciuria
- Chronic disorders:
  — congenital heart disease
  — juvenile arthritis
  — liver disease
  — cystic fibrosis
- Immobilisation:
  — neuromuscular diseases
  — muscular dystrophies
  — paralysis
- Endocrine:
  — Cushing's syndrome
  — thyrotoxicosis
- Nutritional:
  — coeliac disease
  — anorexia
- Drug effects
  — steroids
  — anticonvulsants
  — cytotoxic drugs
- Others:
  — idiopathic juvenile osteoporosis
  — localised osteoporosis – transient osteoporosis of the hip, algodystrophy

---

Idiopathic juvenile osteoporosis presents prepubertally with bone pain, spinal deformity and allied fragility fractures. The diagnosis and investigation of children with osteoporosis is usually within the remit of a specialist bone clinic.

OSTEOPOROSIS OF PREGNANCY

Bone mass may fall in the early months of pregnancy followed by a gain towards term. Lactation may also result in loss of bone mass. These normal physiological changes may coincide with vertebral fracture, usually in the last trimester of pregnancy. Fortunately, recurrence of such fractures is rare in subsequent pregnancies.[12]

4.13 What is the role of guidelines in the management of osteoporosis?

As in so many other areas of medicine, guidelines are available for the management of osteoporosis. The most useful are listed in *Table 4.2,*

TABLE 4.2 Guidelines and allied resources for the management of osteoporosis

Year	Title	Source
1994	Advisory group report on osteoporosis	DOH
1994	Assessment of fracture risk and its application to screening postmenopausal osteoporosis (WHO Technical Report Series)	WHO
1998	Strategy for osteoporosis (Health Service Circular 124)	DOH
1998	Quick reference: primary care guide on the prevention and treatment of osteoporosis	DOH
1998	Preventing accidents caused by osteoporosis (Local Health Actions Sheet)	DOH
1998	Nutrition and bone health: with particular reference to calcium and vitamin D	DOH
1999	Minimum standard guidelines in osteoporosis	PCR
1999	Osteoporosis: clinical guidelines for prevention and treatment	RCP
2000	Update on pharmacological interventions and an algorithm for management	RCP/BTS
2000	Use of bone mineral density in primary care	*
2000	Developing clinical practice guidelines for bone mineral density measurement and osteoporosis management	**
2001	Primary care service strategy for falls and osteoporosis	NOS
2002	Guidelines for the prevention and treatment of glucocorticoid induced osteoporosis	RCP/NOS/BTS
2002	Guidelines for the provision of a clinical bone densitometry service	NOS

BTS, Bone and Tooth Society of Great Britain, London; DOH, Department of Health, London; NOS, National Osteoporosis Society, Bath; PCR, Primary Care Rheumatology Society, Northallerton, North Yorkshire; RCP, Royal College of Physicians, London; WHO, World Health Organization, Geneva.

* Brown P A, p 171–198; ** Hughes R A, p 121–145. Both * and ** in: Fordham J N (ed) Manual of bone densitometry measurements, an aid to the interpretation of bone densitometry measurements in the clinical setting. Springer, London.

together with other resource material. Of these, the Primary Care Rheumatology Society (PCR) guidelines – *Minimum Standard Guidelines in Osteoporosis* – were specifically designed for primary care use. The Royal College of Physicians (RCP) guidelines are evidence-based and should be used as the mainstay of osteoporosis management in the UK. The appended algorithm demonstrates the main groups to be investigated and the appropriate management action. The take-up of such guidelines will depend on local interest and ownership of such tools – influenced by government targets. Osteoporosis does not figure strongly in current targets, but is included in the UK's National Service Framework for Older People which supports the case finding approach advocated by the RCP as well as emphasising the need for the management of other contributing components to fracture risk which are mainly fall related.

Other sources of help include the National Osteoporosis Society document *Primary Care Strategy for Falls and Osteoporosis* which provides a useful resource for GPs to enable them to help develop such services. It includes evidence for the cost effectiveness of the case finding strategy and advice on service commissioning and clinical governance. The need for lead clinicians to be identified in both primary and secondary care is emphasised to help set standards to encourage the development of integrated services covering both primary and secondary care.

PATIENT QUESTIONS

4.14   How might I know that I have or may be at risk of osteoporosis?

There are a number of lifestyle and medical conditions associated with increased risk of osteoporosis. It is important to realise that single risk factors apply to groups of patients with such risk factors and it is impossible to be certain that an individual has osteoporosis based purely on the use of risk factors. To confirm the presence or otherwise of osteoporosis in those at risk, it is necessary to have confirmatory evidence such as bone densitometry measurements usually taken at the hip or spine.

4.15   Do risk factor questionnaires have a role?

Risk factor questionnaires encapsulate known risk factors and can be used to identify those who may have osteoporosis. One such example is the 'One-minute osteoporosis risk test' (*see below*) which has been developed by the International Osteoporosis Foundation. Patients who answer 'yes' to any of the questions may be at risk of fracture. However, the predictability of this tool (and others like it) is not good enough to reliably identify patients with osteoporosis. The next step should be to perform bone densitometry to confirm or refute the presence of the condition.

The one-minute osteoporosis risk test

This simple checklist can provide an indication of whether you should ask your doctor for additional tests, particularly a bone density scan. Only a doctor can perform the necessary tests to find out whether you have osteoporosis, and this checklist is not a substitute for a complete physical examination.

- Have either of your parents broken a hip after a minor bump or fall?
  YES/NO
- Have you broken a bone after a minor bump or fall?
  YES/NO
- Did you undergo the menopause before the age of 45?
  YES/NO
- Have you taken corticosteroid tablets (cortisone, prednisolone, etc.) for more than 6 months?
  YES/NO
- Have you lost more than 5 cm in height?
  YES/NO
- Have your periods ever stopped for 12 months or more for reasons other than pregnancy or the menopause?
  YES/NO
- Do you regularly drink heavily?
  YES/NO
- Do you suffer frequently from diarrhoea (caused by problems such as coeliac disease or Crohn's disease)?
  YES/NO

If you answered 'yes' to any of these questions, you may be at risk of osteoporosis. It is recommended that you consult your doctor who will advise whether further tests are necessary. Take this checklist with you. You may wish to contact one of the osteoporosis societies listed in *Appendix 1* for further information, including details of any local group.

4.16   What are the early warning signs of osteoporosis?

- *A fracture after a minor fall* – This is also known as a fragility fracture (e.g. a wrist or hip fracture).
- *Height loss* – Because bone is lost from the spine this causes weakening and may lead to collapse of vertebrae with consequent loss of height. This is a common feature of osteoporosis, particularly in women in the seventh and eighth decades of life. This may be associated with a curvature (kyphosis) or a twist of the spine (scoliosis). Loss of height may be first detected by women by an apparent lowering of the hemline. Men may notice apparent 'movement' of the waistband upwards.

■ *Back pain* – Episodes of severe back pain lasting for several weeks is suggestive of spinal fracture. Often such back pain is followed by more chronic pain. However, although back pain is a common feature in osteoporosis, there are also other causes of back pain (e.g. due to degeneration of the discs and joints in the back). Such changes can give rise to deformities similar to those seen in osteoporotic patients. An X-ray may help a doctor to elucidate the cause of back pain and the associated deformities.

4.17 What other risk factors for fractures are important?

Although bone density is an important indicator of the likelihood of fracture, there are other factors which independently influence the risk of fracture, notably falls. The risk of falling is greatest in the elderly. It is important to highlight such factors and correct them if possible. Studies of patients who have had hip fractures show that there are a number of factors which independently increase the risk of fracture.

The risk of fracture is increased particularly in those who are over 70, housebound, or in a nursing home. Those who have several risk factors are at particular risk. Some of the risk factors relate to physical fitness and muscular strength, which are obviously related to the risk of falling. Equally relevant is poor vision. Some risks relate to genetic factors, such as a maternal history of fracture. The risk of hip fracture is greatest in the older population, many of whom have, not only low bone density, but also an increased risk of falls. It is important for nursing staff, carers and doctors to be aware of such factors in order to initiate preventative strategies to reduce the risk of fracture.

4.18 How is the diagnosis confirmed?

The normal test for confirming osteoporosis is the use of DXA – dual energy X-ray absorptiometry. These tests are usually requested by a primary care physician/general practitioner once the risk of osteoporosis has been raised. The diagnosis of osteoporosis is based on World Health Organization definitions (*see Table 1.1*, p. 2).

4.19 What other investigations may be carried out?

Once the diagnosis of osteoporosis is confirmed, your GP will wish to discuss the results and to uncover any medical conditions which may be relevant. Physical examination is usually necessary and may give clues to the presence of osteoporosis such as loss of height or curvature of the spine (kyphosis). The cause of osteoporosis may be obvious, such as an early menopause or steroid treatment, in which case other tests may not be necessary. An X-ray of the back may be carried out for signs of height loss or stooping. Your GP may arrange blood tests to detect conditions which may present with osteoporosis. The importance of such tests is that detection and treatment of an underlying cause of osteoporosis – such as reduced absorption of calcium by the gut due to coeliac disease and its subsequent treatment – may go some way to correcting bone loss and reducing the risk of fracture. The tests usually carried out include tests to assess bone activity and levels of the female and male hormones oestrogen and testosterone. In addition to a series of standard tests, there are other more specialised tests which may be needed in particular groups of patients.

In general, the majority of patients with osteoporosis can be investigated and managed by their GP. However, there are groups of patients who will need to be referred to a specialist centre. These include children, male patients and patients with rarer conditions such as osteogenesis imperfecta where specialised management may be necessary.

4.20   Which groups in society are at greatest risk of osteoporosis?

As is discussed elsewhere (*see Ch. 10*), the risk of osteoporosis and the risk of falls increases in the elderly. Patients with such risk factors are commonly found in nursing homes. It is important that a fracture risk assessment is carried out on admission to a nursing home. This should take the form of a review of any risk factors, especially those relating to the liability to fall. At present such assessments are not routinely carried out, and the opportunity of preventing fractures is missed. Since the risk of fracture is greatest in the time shortly after admission to the nursing home – reflecting the disorientating effect of a new environment – greater awareness of this avoidable catastrophe is necessary. Patients in nursing homes may be relatively isolated from routine medical review and the responsibility therefore is on nursing staff and other carers to carry out such appraisals at the time of admission.

Use of bone densitometry and other techniques in the diagnosis and management of osteoporosis

5

5.1   What is the purpose of bone densitometry?

- *The diagnosis of osteoporosis* – The World Health Organization definition of osteoporosis uses T scores, i.e. standard deviation measurements of less than –2.5 below the peak bone density or bone mass of young adults. This level was selected since it identifies approximately 30% of postmenopausal women as at risk of osteoporosis – approximately the same proportion as is found to have fractures in this group. The measurements are taken at the lumbar spine, hip and sometimes forearm. The definition is site, sex and technique dependent and therefore not applicable to other techniques, or other measurement sites.
- *For fracture prediction* – Absolute measurements of bone density presented in standard deviation units from the age and sex matched mean values (Z scores) enable clinicians to relate the risk of fracture to the peer group of the patient, i.e. the relative risk of fracture of an individual can be assigned.
- *To define levels of intervention* – Although the WHO criteria were not intended to define intervention thresholds, in practice – largely as a result of the use of such thresholds in drug trials – intervention is often based on the T score measurement. In the UK, the Royal College of Physicians' recommendations for the management of osteoporosis define interventions in terms of T scores groupings.
- *To monitor changes of bone density with time* – Whilst serial measurement of bone density to assess the effectiveness of treatments is not strictly validated in practice, repeat measurements of bone density of patients receiving treatment are sometimes used for this purpose.

5.2   How are bone density measurements used in clinical practice?

Although it is impossible to clearly define *all* patients who will have fractures on the basis of bone mineral density (BMD) measurements alone, their use is justified on the basis that the predictive value is sufficiently strong to categorise patients at greatest risk of fracture. The use of BMD measurements as a risk factor for fracture is analogous to the use of hypertension to predict stroke, hypercholesterolaemia to predict myocardial infarction or hyperuricaemia to predict arthritis (*Table 5.1*). Obviously, the usefulness of risk factors is dependent on the strength of association with the clinical outcome. The evidence suggests that the gradient of risk of fracture with BMD measurement is greater than that for serum cholesterol or high blood pressure in the prediction of ischaemic heart disease in men

TABLE 5.1 Use of risk factors to predict disease

Risk factor	Disease	Clinical expression
Low bone mineral density	Osteoporosis	Fracture
Hypercholesterolaemia	Ischaemic heart disease	Myocardial infarction
Hyperuricaemia	Gout	Gouty arthritis

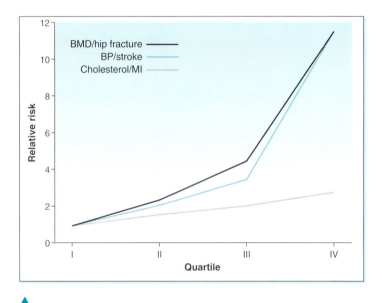

▲

Fig. 5.1 Relative risk of clinical outcomes according to measurement of risk factors categorised by quartiles. Those in the lowest quartile are accorded a risk factor of 1.0. The 25% of the population with the lowest bone mineral density (BMD) has a greater than 10-fold increase in hip fracture risk. BMD measurements perform as well as measurements of blood pressure (BP) to predict stroke, and better than serum cholesterol to predict myocardial infarction (MI) in men. (From Cooper & Aihie[1], by permission of Oxford University Press)

(*Fig. 5.1*). As is the case for blood pressure measurement to predict stroke, BMD measurements have high specificity, but low sensitivity (*see Q. 5.4*).

5.3 What is the predictive value of BMD for fractures?

Prospective studies have shown that BMD measurements predict the risk of fractures. There is a doubling of fracture risk for every standard deviation drop in BMD from the population mean. As can be seen from *Table 5.2*, a

TABLE 5.2 Relative risk of fracture for 1 SD decrease in BMD below the age-adjusted mean (From Marshall et al.[2])

Site of measurement	Forearm fracture	Hip fracture	Vertebral fracture	All fractures
Ultradistal radius	1.7 (1.4–2.0)	1.8 (1.4–2.2)	1.7 (1.4–2.1)	1.4 (1.3–1.6)
Hip	1.4 (1.4–1.6)	2.6 (2.0–3.5)	1.8 (1.1–2.7)	1.6 (1.4–1.8)
Lumbar spine	1.5 (1.3–1.8)	1.6 (1.2–2.2)	2.3 (1.9–2.8)	1.5 (1.4–1.7)
Calcaneus	1.6	2.0	2.4	1.5
Distal radius	1.8	2.1	2.2	1.5

lower gradient of risk is seen with measurements taken at peripheral sites compared with central or axial sites. The greatest predictive value for fracture is found where the measurement is made at the site of potential fracture. The risk of fracture will depend on current BMD, the rate of bone loss and life expectancy.

Relative risk (RR) of fractures is expressed as standard deviation units and as discussed shows a doubling of risk for each standard deviation decline. The effect on fracture risk is exponential such that a patient with a standard deviation decrease has a doubling of fracture risk, i.e. a Z score of $-1 = RR \times 2$, whereas -3 standard deviations (-3 Z) results in an eightfold increased risk of fracture ($Z = -3$ RR $= 8$).

Lifetime fracture risk (LFR) is a method by which a predictive value is given to estimate the fracture risk for an individual taking account of life expectancy, age specific rate of bone loss and specific fracture incidence rates at the site measured. This is calculated by summating the annual fracture risk for each of the expected years of life remaining.

5.4 What do the prospective studies of fracture risk tell us?

Studies have helped clarify the picture regarding several important points: all BMD measurements, regardless of their site, give predictive value of fracture risk. Site specific measurements are of most use in predicting the common clinical fractures.

BMD has high specificity but low sensitivity. This means that a negative test is indicative of a low risk of fracture; low sensitivity in this case means that a significant proportion (50%) of fractures occur in subjects who do not have osteoporosis. This is one of the reasons why population screening is not an appropriate use of the technique, rather a case finding strategy is advocated, i.e. subjects at greater risk of osteoporosis are 'selected' for bone density measurements.

Although BMD is a strong risk factor for fractures, other measurements, such as those derived from ultrasound techniques are also important in predicting fracture. In the EPIDOS study[3] calcaneal ultrasound was used and found to predict increased risk of hip fracture with equivalent power of hip dual energy X-ray absorptiometry (DXA).

The Study of Osteoporotic Fractures (SOF)[4] has shed light on the effects of risk factors other than low BMD on the risk of hip fractures (*Fig. 5.2*). This has shown that combinations of risk factors increase the RR of fracture.

5.5 Where and how is bone density usually measured in the skeleton?

Bone density is usually measured at the lumbar spine, the measurement being taken in the anteroposterior (AP) dimension. Spinal BMD reflects the bone density of the vertebral body as well as the spinous processes and spinal arches. The measurement is thus a composite of cancellous (largely vertebral body) as well as cortical bone (the arch and spinous processes). The second site routinely measured is the femoral neck or the total hip. The measurements are presented as areal values derived from the dimensions of the sites. The results are not therefore true volumetric density values.

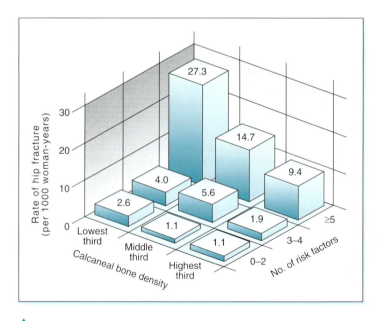

▲

Fig. 5.2 Annual risk of hip fractures relative to age specific heel bone density and the number of risk factors. (From Cummings et al.[4])

Each site value can be presented in absolute measurements, i.e. g/cm^2, T scores, or age related standard deviation units – Z scores. Results can also be represented as a percentage of the mean result for the age- and sex-matched population or as centiles.

The technique of measurement is based on dual X-ray absorptiometry (DXA) (*Figs 5.3–5.5*). This is the standard method in current use. This technique has superseded earlier techniques such as photon absorptiometry which were based on radionuclide sources of photons rather than X-rays.

5.6 Should DXA be used to monitor treatment and if so, how often?

Repeat bone densitometry measurement is used by some in order to assess the effect of treatments and has a secondary benefit in encouraging compliance. Although widespread, this practice is subject to question:

■ The precision of the technique is insufficient to enable short term effects in patients. Longer intervals are needed to ensure that the measured difference is greater than the error of the measurement. In practice therefore, repeat measurements are not usually undertaken more frequently than every 2 years.

■ Age related bone loss in postmenopausal women may average 2% so that longer intervals may be needed to detect any positive effect on bone density.

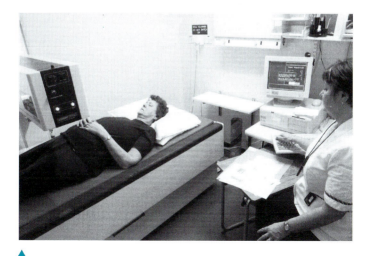

▲

Fig. 5.3 DXA scanning of right hip.

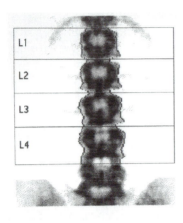
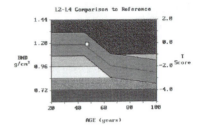

Region	BMD g/cm²	Young-Adult %	T	Age-Matched %	Z
L1	1.088	96	−0.3	99	−0.1
L2	1.170	98	−0.2	100	0.0
L3	1.241	103	0.3	106	0.6
L4	1.164	97	−0.3	100	0.0
L2-L4	1.191	99	−0.1	102	0.2

▲

Fig. 5.4 DXA scan of lumbar spine. The average of the L2/L3/L4 results is calculated and represented as an absolute measurement or as a T score (1.191 g/cm² or −0.1, respectively).

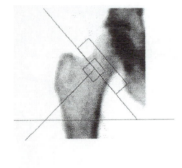
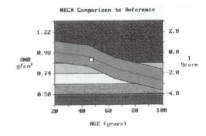

Region	BMD g/cm²	Young-Adult %	T	Age-Matched %	Z
NECK	0.899	92	−0.7	97	−0.2
WARDS	0.768	84	−1.1	94	−0.4
TROCH	0.781	99	−0.1	101	0.1
SHAFT	0.981	−	−	−	−
TOTAL	0.895	90	−0.9	93	−0.6

▲

Fig. 5.5 DXA scan of right hip. Results are represented as absolute measurements or T scores at femoral neck, Ward's triangle, trochanter or total hip.

■ Large drug trials have shown significant variability in the response of individuals within the population treated – 'non-responders' and 'responders'. Such studies have also illustrated the regression to the mean phenomenon, i.e. those patients with the largest loss of bone in the first year of treatment show the greatest gain in the second year. Although this is a statistical quirk, it has added to the doubts about the usefulness of repeat DXA measurements in assessing effectiveness of treatment.

■ The long interval between measurements makes them less clinically useful in aiding compliance. In this regard, bone markers may ultimately be of more use.

Notwithstanding these caveats, repeat bone densitometry is likely to continue to be used to monitor compliance and effectiveness of treatments until such time as alternatives such as bone markers become readily available.

5.7   What other techniques may be used?

■ *Quantitative computed tomography* (QCT) – This offers true volumetric density measurements and can be applied to peripheral and spinal sites. Femoral BMD measurement may be possible using spiral CT scanning. Because of the ability to scan specific regions within individual bones, it is possible to select the cancellous component which is mainly susceptible to osteoporotic changes. Despite this advantage, the use of QCT is relatively limited for the reasons indicated in *Table 5.3*.

■ *Magnetic resonance imaging* (MRI) – This offers the ability to assess the microarchitecture of bone. Trabecular thickness, numbers of trabeculae and the connectivity of trabeculae can be measured using this technique. These measurements relate to the integrity of bone which is an important factor in determining bone strength. Thus changes in bone structure in response to interventions may be detectable. At the moment, such techniques are limited to research and their general applicability is unlikely to be great in view of the cost and difficulties in representing the results of complex measurements.

■ *Ultrasound-based techniques* – Numerous devices based on ultrasonic transmission through bone have been in use since the early 1980s. Advantages of this methodology include portability of the devices, speed of measurement and lack of irradiation. Various modalities of ultrasound transmission through bone have been shown to be related to fracture risk. Such measurements include speed of sound (SOS) and broadband ultrasonic attenuation (BBUA). Indices derived from these measurements include stiffness and qualitative ultrasound index (QUI). These measurements are not of bone density per se, but relate to the connectivity of bone and may give information about the qualitative features of bone as well as reflecting the amount of bone present.

■ *Digital radiogrammetry* – This is based on the analysis of X-ray films; the use of such techniques is undergoing evaluation.

TABLE 5.3 Techniques used in measurement of bone mass

Technique	Site	Cancellous bone (%)	Accuracy (%)	Precision (%)	Scan time (min)	Micro μSv	Comments
DXA	Lumbar spine	50	5–8	1–3	10	1	Gold standard method; central and appendicular sites; low irradiation dose; costly
	Femur	40	5–8	1–2	10	1	Offers several sites for scanning
	Forearm	40	2–5	1–2	10	<1	Hip results strongly predictive of fracture
	Total body	20	1–2	1	20	3	Can be used to detect vertebral abnormalities and bone size
SxA/pDXA	Forearm – distal	5	2.5	1–2	10	<1	Low irradiation dose
	Forearm – ultradistal	40	2.5	1–2	10	<1	Low cost; portable
	Os calcis	95	2.5	1–2	5	<1	Lower fracture predictability than axial sites
QCT	Lumbar spine	100	3–6	2–4	15	60	True volumetric density; cancellous site measurement; higher radiation dose, higher costs; not applicable to femur; slow
QUS	Os calcis Tibia Patella Phalanges	95		3–5	1–5	0	No irradiation; good fracture prediction in those > 65 years; small, cheap, portable devices; many different techniques; poor costs correlation, poor precision

Accuracy, ability to give the same result as another method on the same object; precision, the reproducibility of results from the same object. DXA, dual energy X-ray absorptiometry; QCT, quantitative computed tomography; QUS, quantitative ultrasound; SxA/pDXA, single X-ray absorptiometry/peripheral scanner based on dual energy X-ray absorptiometry.

5.8   Why are spinal and hip sites used to measure bone density?

The common clinically important fracture sites are the vertebrae, femoral neck and forearm. These are cancellous rich sites which reflect the changes in bone density that occur in osteoporosis. As discussed, studies of the value of bone density at various sites in the skeleton have shown that the power of fracture prediction increases when the bone density measurement is made at the site of potential fracture. Thus, the relative risk of fracture for a standard deviation decrease in bone density at the hip is 2.6 whereas the relative risk of hip fracture when bone density is measured at the lumbar spine, forearm and os calcis ranges from 1.6 to 2.1 (*see Table 5.2*). The calcaneal site is the exception to this general rule with relatively good predictive power for vertebral fractures (–2.4 RR) and hip (–2 RR), the predictive power being similar to measurements made at the spine and hip.

5.9   Which other sites can be measured?

■ *Total body* – Such measurements are used in juveniles where, because of small body size, the usual sites cannot be used. The technique usually allows additional information about body composition to be measured at the same 'sitting'.

■ *Forearm* – This site is valuable in predicting forearm–Colles fractures especially in women of 55–60 and older. The measurement is made at the distal radius and ulna and requires accurate positioning. The percentage of cancellous bone is 5% at the distal radius and 40% at the ultradistal site.

■ *Calcaneum* – The calcaneum is a cancellous rich site (95%). The site is easily accessible and relatively free of positioning and artefactual errors. It provides good predictive values for fractures of the spine, forearm and hip and has similar predictive powers for hip and spinal fractures as measurements made at these sites.

■ *Lateral spine* – Measurements of the lateral spine are sometimes made where artefacts may interfere with the normal AP scan. These include calcification of the aorta and degenerative changes of the facetal joints and discs. The advantage of lateral scanning, which enables true cancellous rich sites to be scanned, is offset to some degree by the disadvantages of inaccuracies due to difficulties in accurately positioning the subject.

5.10   What are the advantages of axial scanning?

■ These machines offer good precision and accuracy which are particularly important where serial measurements are being used to gauge the effectiveness of treatment.

■ The measurements at the central as opposed to the peripheral site are of cancellous rich bone (with the exception of the os calcis).

■ The measurements are undertaken at sites of clinical relevance, i.e. where fractures commonly occur.

■ The effects of most drugs used in osteoporosis have been largely studied at these sites.

■ The predictive power of measurements of bone density at these sites for fracture is higher than where peripheral sites are used.

■ The reference data against which to report results are extensive and well validated compared with the relative paucity of data for peripheral scanning.

5.11 What are the disadvantages of axial scanners?

Because of the large size, expense and cumbersome nature of these devices, they cannot be easily used outside the hospital setting and therefore are not easily applicable to a primary care setting (general practice). Furthermore, they are technician dependent. The scanning times are relatively slow and spinal scans are particularly subject to artefacts in older patients, largely due to degenerative disc disease. (Hip scans are relatively free of such disadvantages.)

5.12 What are the advantages of peripheral scanners?

Peripheral scanners based on DXA (pDXA) offer good precision and accuracy with a reasonable prediction of fractures of the spine and hip, particularly where the os calcis is used. They have the advantages of lower cost, smaller size, portability and rapid scan speed. They are therefore more suited to use in the community setting.

5.13 What are the disadvantages of peripheral scanners?

Osteoporosis is defined in terms of bone mineral mass of the lumbar spine, hip and forearm. Strictly speaking therefore, peripheral measurements can only be used to identify those at risk of fracture rather than to establish the diagnosis of osteoporosis.

Although there is a correlation between pDXA and central DXA sites, this is relatively weak. Therefore, it is not possible to use pDXA to identify patients reliably as osteoporotic at the spine or hip on the basis of a peripheral site reading alone.

■ It has been suggested that these techniques can be used to 'stream' patients into those at greatest risk of osteoporosis, or as definitely normal or intermediate, the intermediate group being referred for axial scanning.[5]

- Since changes in BMD following drug treatments at peripheral sites, especially the forearm, are relatively small, such sites cannot be used to monitor the effects of treatment.[6]
- pDXA devices have limited applicability in premenopausal women, men and children due to the relatively small normal databases available.
- Because of lack of standardisation between scanners, the results cannot be compared between manufacturers. Limited normative data and variability of inclusion and exclusion criteria of different manufacturers, particularly relating to racial mix and children's data, all militate against their indiscriminate use.
- pDXA scanning requires compliance with ionising radiation regulations,[7,8] as do axial DXA devices.

5.14 When and how should pDXA be used?

When there is no access to axial measurements then their use can be justified. However, *their use is to assess fracture risk rather than to diagnose osteoporosis*. The commonly used sites in these circumstances are the forearm and os calcis. *Box 5.1* illustrates the recommendations of an expert group convened by the National Osteoporosis Society.[9] As can be seen, the interventions advised are based on the use of forearm scans. Similar interventions may ultimately be developed for other measurement sites (e.g. the calcaneum).

5.15 What is the predictive value of ultrasound measurements for fractures?

Large studies using ultrasound have shown that speed of sound (SOS) measurement and broadband ultrasonic attenuation (BBUA) predict liability to hip fracture in elderly women.[3,10] Such measurements of the os calcis were carried out using water-based devices. Other 'dry' systems have also been shown to have predictive powers for hip fractures in elderly men and women. Further studies[11,12] have shown the predictive power of ultrasound for Colles fracture in the early postmenopausal years and for any other fractures in the perimenopausal years. Such measurements do not appear to be of use in predicting vertebral fractures.

5.16 Can ultrasound be used to diagnose osteoporosis?

Despite the fact that the measurement of bone density and ultrasound parameters at the same site correlate with each other, these associations are not strong enough to derive true bone density values reliably from ultrasound measurements. Nevertheless, ultrasound does give information about the integrity of bone[12,13] which is related to bone strength.

BOX 5.1 Position statement on the use of peripheral X-ray absorptiometry in the management of osteoporosis (From National Osteoporosis Society[9])

1. Bone mineral density (BMD) measurement by DXA at the lumbar spine and proximal femur remain the current 'gold standard' for the diagnosis of patients with osteoporosis.

2. If axial (lumbar spine and proximal femur) BMD measurements are not available, a bone mineral density measurement in a peripheral skeletal site (forearm or calcaneus) can be used to predict fracture risk.

3. Intervention is recommended as follows:
   - if the forearm T-score is less than –2.5, treatment is recommended, especially if other major risk factors for osteoporosis and/or fractures are present.
   - if the forearm T-score lies between –1 and –2.5 then lumbar spine and proximal femur BMD measurement by DXA should be performed.
   - if the forearm T-score is greater than –1.0, and no low trauma fractures are present, then no further treatment is required, and the patient should be reassured that his/her risk of fracture is low.

4. The lumbar spine is the best site for monitoring the efficacy of treatment.

5. The distal forearm site (predominantly cortical bone) is not sufficiently sensitive to monitor changes in BMD with time and treatment. If change in bone mineral density is to be monitored, patients who initially have had forearm bone density measurements will need referral for a DXA at the spine and/or hip before commencing therapy.

6. The calcaneus, which is predominantly trabecular bone (90–95%), has the potential for monitoring change. However, longitudinal studies using newer calcaneal scanning devices have not yet been reported.

7. This advice relates principally to the diagnosis of fracture risk and osteoporosis is postmenopausal women in clinical practice; research on which to base advice for such diagnosis in premenopausal women and men is relatively scanty, and these peripheral techniques do not yet have a clearly defined role in clinical practice in children.

8. All peripheral X-ray devices must be operated by trained staff, to ensure adequate quality control and reproducible results. Their operation should comply with legislation governing the use of ionising radiation. Interpretation of the results must be provided by an experienced physician, with specific knowledge of osteoporosis and its management.

The role of ultrasound techniques in the management of osteoporosis is summarised in the position statement of the National Osteoporosis Society[14] (*Box 5.2*). In essence, the use of this technique should be restricted to postmenopausal women. When low values of quantitative ultrasound (QUS) are found then such patients should be referred for DXA to confirm or refute the diagnosis of osteoporosis; where other strong risk factors (e.g. low trauma fracture) are present then preventative treatment may be used.

5.17 Can ultrasound be used to screen the population for axial bone densitometry?

Current opinion suggests that ultrasound techniques are better than clinical risk factors in defining women at risk of low bone mass.[15,16] However, there is insufficient evidence at the moment to justify the use of ultrasound as a

---

BOX 5.2 Position statement on the use of quantitative ultrasound in the management of osteoporosis (From National Osteoporosis Society[14])

1. As quantitative ultrasound (QUS) does not measure bone mineral content or density directly, it cannot be used to diagnose osteoporosis as currently defined by bone mineral content (BMC) or bone mineral density (BMD) assessment.
2. Low QUS is an independent risk factor for future osteoporotic fracture in postmenopausal women.
3. Low QUS parameters are stronger predictors of low bone mass than clinical risk factors; individuals found to have low QUS parameters (as defined by machine-specific normative data) may *either*

   ■ be referred for confirmation of the diagnosis by axial (preferably hip) BMD measurement *or*
   ■ be advised to receive preventative therapy if other strong clinical risk factors are present.

4. In most cases QUS measurements cannot be used to monitor bone loss or assess response to therapy in an individual patient.
5. At present the use of QUS for assessment of bone mass in children, premenopausal women and men for clinical care purposes is not recommended.
6. Trained staff must operate all QUS devices and they should be able to demonstrate precision of measurement within the manufacturer's specification. An experienced physician with specific knowledge of osteoporosis and its management must interpret results.

screening tool in the general population to select patients for axial bone densitometry.

5.18 Can ultrasound be used to target patients for therapy?

Ultrasound is used to define patients at risk of fracture. However, different machines – even using the same measurement techniques – identify different subjects. In addition, therapeutic studies of the effect of anti-resorptive drugs have been based on selection by bone density measurement rather than by ultrasound. Therefore, ultrasound methods should not be used routinely to direct patients to drug treatments with the exception as discussed in *Question 5.16*.

Therefore, if one is to use ultrasound for identifying patients to treat, then this should be followed up by an axial bone densitometry measurement, where available, to confirm or refute the diagnosis of osteoporosis. Inevitably this will result in some patients being identified by ultrasound as at risk of fracture who do not have low bone density.

5.19 Can ultrasound be used to monitor the effects of drugs?

Ultrasound measurements are relatively imprecise and since the effects of drugs may be small, it is unlikely that the technique can reliably detect treatment effects (i.e. the effect of the treatment on the bone measurement must be greater than the error or the measurement itself). Additionally there are few data about changes in ultrasound measurement following drug treatment. These devices should therefore not be used in this context.

5.20 What are bone markers?

Bone markers are biochemical markers of bone turnover. Changes in their level reflect bone formation and remodelling (*Table 5.4*). They are categorised into two groups:

1. *Bone formation markers* – These include alkaline phosphatase and osteocalcin which are produced by osteoblasts
2. *Bone resorption markers* – Osteoclasts secrete acid phosphatase, hydroxyproline and hydroxylysine glycosides which results in increased excretion of type I collagen breakdown products – hydroxyproline and collagen crosslinks – which can be measured in the urine.

Biochemical markers have largely replaced the need for calcium balance studies. They are non-invasive, relatively cheap and can be used repeatedly. They also reflect changes throughout the skeleton.

> **TABLE 5.4 The range of biochemical markers proposed for use in the assessment of bone turnover. (Modified from Eastell & Price[17], further modified from Blumsohn & Eastell 1997 Ann Clin Biochem 34:449–459)**
>
> | Formation | Resorption |
> |---|---|
> | Serum | Urine |
> | — total alkaline phosphatase | — pyridinoline (total or free) |
> | — bone alkaline phosphatase | — deoxypyridinoline (total or free) |
> | — osteocalcin | — N-telopeptide (NTX) |
> | — procollagen-1-N-peptide (PINP) | — C-telopeptide (Crosslaps, CTX) |
> | — procollagen-1-C-peptide (PICP) | |
> | | Serum |
> | | — tartrate resistant acid phosphatase Type 56 |
> | | — C-telopeptide (CTX) |

5.21 What are the advantages of bone markers?

■ When used to monitor response, they can give early evidence of the effect of treatment whereas assessing response by bone densitometry requires a longer interval, usually of at least 2 years.

■ Responses to treatment are significant and occur soon after treatment is started. Characteristically resorption markers are suppressed by about 50% with the first 3 months of treatment. The extent of such changes is, to some degree, related to the drug used.

5.22 Can bone markers be used to predict and monitor response to therapy?

As bone markers reflect bone turnover, they may be used in this manner. Drugs such as bisphosphonates, hormone replacement therapy (HRT) and calcitriol reduce markers of bone resorption. Bone formation markers decrease more slowly with treatment. Monitoring changes in bone markers can therefore give surrogate evidence of drug compliance and efficacy. Their use in monitoring therapy is subject to the problems of variability discussed below. There is also uncertainty as to whether individual changes in such markers predict long term effects on bone density and fracture risk.

5.23 What are the disadvantages of bone markers?

Bone markers have a number of disadvantages, mainly due to variability of measurement. The causes include circadian variation (maximal bone resorption occurs at night) and day to day variability (up to 20% for resorption markers). They are also subject to variability in relation to the menstrual cycle, bone formation being greater in luteal rather than in the follicular phase of menstruation. There are also seasonal changes. Their levels are increased after fractures.

Other caveats include:

- Changes in bone turnover are relatively small in comparison to the large variability of bone markers.
- There are high levels of bone turnover at times of peak bone growth such as during adolescence.
- They reflect other disorders of bone metabolism such as hyperparathyroidism and osteomalacia.

5.24 What other uses for bone markers are there?

Bone markers can also predict bone loss. Because high turnover of bone at the menopause may be associated with increased bone loss, it has been suggested that bone markers could be used on an individual basis in early menopausal women in conjunction with BMD measurement, to predict low bone density and fracture risk later in life. At present the evidence is not strong enough to suggest their use on such a basis. Their use is largely confined to regional laboratories and specialised bone clinics.

5.25 What is the role of biochemical markers in the prediction of fracture risk?

In older women, high bone resorption markers predict a greater risk of hip fracture.

5.26 Can bone markers be used to diagnose osteoporosis?

Although bone resorption markers may be elevated in patients with osteoporosis, there is a poor correlation between bone marker levels and BMD results. Just as ultrasound cannot be used to diagnose osteoporosis, bone markers cannot be used in this way either. Nor is there current evidence at present to validate the use of bone markers as pre-screening tools prior to bone density measurement.

5.27 Where can I obtain further information about the use of bone markers?

Eastell & Bainbridge[18] provide an excellent review of this subject.

PATIENT QUESTIONS

5.28 Should I have a bone density scan?

If you have any risk factors for osteoporosis, as listed below, then it is advisable to discuss with your primary care physician/general practitioner the question of bone density measurement. Although risk factors for osteoporosis are well known, they are not in themselves sufficiently reliable to establish the diagnosis. In some cases, it is not necessary to have bone measurements carried out since the likelihood may already be very high. This is the case in elderly men or women who have sustained a particular type of fracture, i.e. a fracture of the hip, forearm or vertebra. Similarly, the incidence of osteoporosis increases steeply in old age and it is very likely that an old person with a fracture will have osteoporosis.

Common risk factors for osteoporosis include:

- early menopause (before the age of 45)
- missed periods (for 6 months)
- hysterectomy or oophorectomy (removal of ovaries and uterus)
- use of steroids
- maternal history of hip fracture or vertebral fracture
- malabsorption (e.g. Crohn's disease or ulcerative colitis, gastric surgery)
- alcohol excess
- smoking
- thinness
- immobility
- fracture.

5.29 Is bone densitometry always necessary?

Often the clinical setting will make it evident that a patient has an osteoporosis related fracture, for example an elderly lady falling at home with a history of previous spinal fracture, spinal deformity or height loss, or in whom X-rays have shown spinal fractures. In these situations, the usefulness of bone density is slight.

Similarly, women after the menopause who have already elected to take HRT do not routinely require bone density measurements unless they are contemplating stopping treatment. Where the decision to treat a patient has already been taken there is little point in performing bone densitometry.

5.30 If I am already using HRT or another agent for the treatment of osteoporosis, should I have a scan?

There is usually no need to have a bone density scan if a person is already taking such treatments. For those contemplating stopping treatment, be that HRT or a bisphosphonate, then it may be useful to have a bone density measurement since if this is low, then continued treatment or an alternative treatment may be appropriate.

5.31   What is the basis of the scan and what will it tell me?

Bone densitometry (or DXA) is an X-ray-based method by which the density of bones is deduced by the amount of X-ray that pass through the bones scanned. From this, it is possible to measure the bone in the spine or hip. By comparison with normal values in the population, it is possible to assess the risk of fracture. Readings are based on the T score – this is a measurement compared to the peak bone density of young adults. Since treatments are most effective in those patients with the lowest bone density, it is important to use these results in order to target those people most likely to benefit from treatment.

5.32   What does the measurement entail?

DXA does not involve undressing or going into a tunnel or confined space – unlike an MRI or CT examination. The measurements are undertaken at the hip and spinal sites and involve lying still for about 10 minutes. In some circumstances, measurements at the forearm or heel may be undertaken.

5.33   Should bone densitometry measurements be repeated?

Your doctor may advise that a repeat DXA measurement be undertaken to assess the effect of the treatment on bones. Because the effects of drugs on bone are slow, the usual time for a repeat bone measurement is 2 years after the previous measurement.

5.34   What other methods are sometimes used?

Ultrasound-based methods rely on the speed of transmission of sound through bone. These measurements have been shown to predict hip fracture risk particularly for elderly men and women and wrist fractures in early postmenopausal women. The methods however do not measure bone density as does DXA and it is not possible to diagnose osteoporosis using such devices. They are used to indicate the liability of fractures when access to DXA scans is not possible.

5.35   What is the role of urine tests in the diagnosis of osteoporosis?

These tests are based on the use of markers of bone production and the breakdown products of bone in urine and blood. When bone is being lost from the skeleton, increased breakdown products of bone occur. Measurements of these products are used in some hospital practices to monitor the response of patients to drugs and to assess compliance, i.e. to ensure that patients are taking the drug correctly. Because there is a weak link between such measurements and bone density, and because osteoporosis is only diagnosable by use of bone density measurements, they cannot be used to confirm osteoporosis. The role of these tests is being evaluated internationally; they may have an ultimate use in identifying patients at risk of fracture, and in the regular monitoring of drug treatment as an additional aid to doctors.

Health economics in osteoporosis

6

6.1 What different tools are used to assess the effectiveness of interventions in osteoporosis?

Epidemiological data gathered about the number of fractures occurring in populations, together with analysis of the cost of management in both medical and societal terms, can be employed to assess their financial burden. This includes analysis of the impact on quality of life (*Table 6.1*). Economic models can then be applied to questions such as: Do bone densitometry scans or other screening methods (e.g. ultrasound techniques or bone markers) provide value for money in terms of detection of patients at risk of fractures? Similarly, where there are 'competing' prevention or treatment options available, such as HRT or bisphosphonates, selective (o)estrogen receptor modulators (SERMs) etc., then the question of the optimal choice for particular patients can be addressed.

Such evaluations may be on the basis of *cost minimisation* in which agents are compared to each other in terms of cost alone. The presumption in this model is that the effectiveness of each intervention will be the same.

Cost benefit analysis is an alternative method by which all the benefits of treatment are translated into financial terms. In practice, it is sometimes difficult to apply such analyses since the value of life and the quality of life are not easily measured in financial terms.

Cost effectiveness takes into account the fact that effectiveness and the risks of different treatments are not usually the same. In this model, the outcomes are interpreted as financial (e.g. cost per fracture prevented). However, again it is not always easy to express outcomes simply in financial terms. Additionally, comparisons of the cost of fractures prevented are different for different fractures (e.g. hip fracture versus vertebral fracture).

Cost utility analysis is used more commonly in the context of fracture prevention and takes into account the numbers of fractures prevented as well as changes in associated morbidity. Quality adjusted life years (QALYs) are used as the units of measurement. Each year of life is valued from 0 (least desirable) to 1 (perfect health).

TABLE 6.1 Types of economic evaluation

Technique	Outcome measured	Unit of value
Cost minimisation	Outcomes assumed identical	
Cost benefit	Effects of alternatives equal	Pounds sterling (£)
Cost effectiveness	Single outcome achieved to variable extent	Life years
Cost utility	Effects of different therapies achieved to different degrees	Quality adjusted life years (QALYs)

6.2   What are the components of the cost of fracture to society?

The costs of hip fracture in the UK have been estimated as approximately £5000 for the direct hospital care of such patients. When the non-hospital costs are taken into account (related to the use of sheltered accommodation, nursing homes, etc.), then costs increase to about £12 000 per year.[1] Costs reduce after the second year of hip fracture to about £7000 per year. The total cost of hip fractures to the UK is estimated at £1728 million per year. These figures, and data from drug trials of anti-fracture efficacy, together with compliance information, provide the basis of health economic modelling used to deduce which drugs provide the best value for money in the particular groups of people at risk of fracture.

6.3   What does health economics tell us about the appropriate use of HRT?

Where such techniques have been applied to the use of HRT, certain assumptions have been made: that the overall reduction in hip fracture risk is about 50%; that there is a modest risk of breast cancer after about 5 years of treatment; and that cardiovascular disease is reduced by 30–50%.

In recent years these assumptions have been challenged, particularly the question of effects on cardiovascular disease which now appear to be adverse rather than beneficial, this being particularly the case in the first year of HRT treatment. The evidence for fracture prevention, although not strong, is still supportive – the Women's Health Initiative (WHI) study[2] confirmed anti-fracture efficacy. The cost of HRT is low relative to other options (*Box 6.1*) and this factor goes some way to negating the cost implications of increased risk of breast cancer and adverse cardiovascular events.

> ### BOX 6.1 The use of HRT in postmenopausal women (From Compston et al.[3])
>
> ■ Cost per quality adjusted life year when oestrogen is used in hysterectomised women compares favourably with other healthcare interventions
> ■ Costs increase considerably when HRT is used for all women at risk
> ■ Targeting of HRT on the basis of fracture risk (using BMD measurement) is more cost effective than treating all women
> ■ Targeting of elderly women (over 65) is more cost effective than treating at the menopause

Targeting women by use of bone densitometry to identify those with lowest bone mineral density appears to be the most cost effective model. HRT is usually prescribed early after the menopause for both climacteric symptoms and in the prevention of osteoporosis. However, HRT has effects on bone density in later life as well. The argument for using HRT in later life is based on the efficacy of this agent at this age and the facts that the risk of breast cancer is less since life expectancy is shorter. Women who use HRT at the menopause and then stop in their sixties have relatively small increases in bone mineral density (BMD) as they subsequently enter the fracture decades. Delaying HRT until the mid-sixties results in increases in BMD similar to those when HRT is given in the early postmenopausal years.[4] Additional benefits of HRT in later life include those on cognitive function and balance.

Notwithstanding these arguments for the use of HRT, especially in women over 65, given the WHI study findings and for other reasons – notably the emotive nature of breast cancer for most women, the attenuation of effect after stopping therapy, and the advent of other treatment options – the use of HRT is likely to decline and the core use of these agents is likely to be the control of menopausal symptoms.

6.4 What is the cost effectiveness of raloxifene?

Data produced by the NHS Research and Development Health Technology Assessment Programme are shown in *Table 6.2*. The modelling of

TABLE 6.2 Annual costs and cost effectiveness of different treatments (From National Osteoporosis Society[5])

Cost (£ per annum)	Agent	Cost at 70 years	Cost at 80 years
2314	Calcitonin	168	124
334	Alendronate	13.3	d-ing
257	Raloxifene[a]	46.4	76.1
163	Bisphosphonates	5.7	d-ing
157	Vitamin D derivatives[a]	36.5	30.1
58	HRT[b]	5.0	d-ing
55	Calcium and vitamin D	d-ing	d-ing
40	Calcium	15.9	16.3

[a]Assumes relative risk + 1 for appendicular fractures, e.g. Colles fracture.
[b]Assumes benefit on coronary heart disease and increased risk of breast cancer.
d-ing = dominating. When comparing two interventions using health economics, one usually dominates the other: that is, as a result of the review, cost efficacy is proven in one case (i.e. the dominating intervention), or that no review is required for it to be clear that one is cheaper and more effective than the other.

raloxifene, which has both anti-fracture efficacy and anti-breast cancer effects, is shown. Anti-fracture efficacy is confined to vertebral fracture reduction and the effect on breast cancer prevention, although adding cost utility, is maximal in women with high, not low bone density.[6] Therefore, since the evidence for efficacy of raloxifene is mainly in those women with low BMD who have a lower likelihood of breast cancer, the added benefit of the drug will be less. By comparison to other treatments, this drug is relatively costly.

6.5 What is the cost effectiveness of bisphosphonates?

The cost effectiveness of these agents is maximal when patients at greatest risk of fracture are selected for treatment. Bone density or ultrasound measurements, combined with other risk factors are most likely to identify those with the greatest risk of fracture. Since hip fractures are the most serious of the common osteoporotic fractures, main attention has been directed at these. The most important risk factors for hip fractures are[7]:

- low body weight (less than 58 kg)
- maternal history or sibling history of hip fracture
- current smoking
- prior fracture since the age of 40
- low BMD of the femur.

These factors can be used to 'target' those most likely to benefit from treatment. Most of the studies of bisphosphonates show that their efficacy in terms of fracture prevention is maximal in those with lowest BMD. This is exemplified by the study of Cummings et al.[8] where alendronate was studied in patients with low BMD but who did not have vertebral fractures; fracture reduction only occurred in those with BMD in the osteoporotic range. Similar findings were found in studies of risedronate. Anti-fracture efficacy of bisphosphonates increases when there are prevalent vertebral fractures.

To summarise, the effectiveness of bisphosphonates is maximal in those with low BMD (T scores of –2 to –2.5), with prevalent vertebral fractures, or in those with low BMD alone.

6.6 What is the cost effectiveness of calcium and vitamin D or calcium alone in the elderly?

Table 6.2 shows that the use of calcium and vitamin D can be justified in both 70 and 80-year-olds with overwhelming cost effectiveness; even calcium alone is cost effective. Models of different strategies in targeting the residents of nursing homes, where hip fracture rates are higher than in the community, show that those with low body weight are most appropriately treated. However, it is now common practice that all residents of nursing homes are offered calcium and vitamin D. The relative cheapness of this combination together with moderate anti-fracture efficacy make this good value for money.

6.7 What are the drawbacks of economic modelling?

Most of the models have used hip fracture prevention as the goal of interventions. Since most drugs have anti-fracture efficacy at other sites, the potential cost efficiency of such agents is likely to be underestimated. However, such gains may be offset by decline in long term efficacy of some drugs, and possible attenuation of efficacy after treatment has stopped. Obviously the usefulness of economic modelling of this kind depends on the validity and completeness of supportive data. Since there are 'gaps' in knowledge in many areas, especially in groups such as men and children, these models cannot be applied in such cases.

6.8 What is the evidence for cost effectiveness of bone densitometry used in case finding?

An estimation of the effects of introducing a bone densitometry service based on certain assumptions (*Box 6.2*) shows that the net cost of each averted hip fracture would be £1374 and a cost per life year saved of £22 558 (*Box 6.3*). If benefits were to continue over 5 years, the costs for hip fracture prevention would average £275 and £4500 per life year saved, respectively.

The cost effectiveness of using bone densitometry improves with greater cost of treatment, i.e. the costs of each averted fracture using densitometry where clinically relevant would be £2887 compared with £8453 if all eligible patients were treated.

BOX 6.2 Indications for bone densitometry (based on European Foundation for Osteoporosis, DOH Advisory Group[9] and RCP Osteoporosis Guidelines Writing Group[10])

- Patients with symptomatic vertebral fractures
- Patients with forearm fractures/radiological osteoporosis
- Women uncertain of continued use of HRT who predicate the use of HRT on the basis of low BMD
- Patients starting on long term high dose corticosteroids

BOX 6.3   Effects of introducing bone densitometry for case finding based on indications in Box 6.2 for a population of 300 000 (From Compston et al.[3])

- 14 Vertebral, 3 forearm, 1 hip fracture prevented per annum
- 1.11 life years saved
- Treatment costs: £7800
- Bone densitometry costs: £38 240
- Net cost per fracture: £1374
- Cost per life year saved: £22 558
- Presumptions for 300 000 population based on 1995 costs:
    - 700–1000 measurements per year
    - 1% annual incidence of axial, vertebral and forearm fractures
    - management costs of £1000 for vertebral and forearm fractures
    - treatments costs of £200 per patient per annum
    - efficacy of 50% reduction in fractures
    - 50% compliance

 PATIENT QUESTIONS

6.9   What is the cost of preventing and treating fractures?

The costs of treating patients with fractures include:

- surgical treatment including the surgeon's time
- materials (e.g. hip replacement)
- rehabilitation
- accommodation in hospital – the so called hotel costs.

These costs, and those additionally incurred by the patient if discharged to a nursing home or residential home (instead of back to their own home), are the obvious costs to the patient and society. The impact of fracture in terms of the quality of life of patients is often significant, especially after a hip fracture when at its worst, death may occur.

When comparing the effects of different treatments, it is important to take into account both financial factors and the effects on quality of life. It is often difficult to ascribe a financial cost to changes in quality of life. In order to get around this difficulty, health economists have developed a measure of the health outcome – quality adjusted life years or QALYs. In this way, measurement of the quality of life on a scale of 0 (least desirable) to 1 (perfect health) can be applied to patients and it is possible to measure the effects of treatments as well as the impact of fractures in both health and quality of life gains. Such analysis helps to direct the use of drugs to those who are most likely to benefit from them.

6.10 How can such measures help doctors in the management of their patients?

Drug treatments for osteoporosis can only be used after they have been proven in clinical trials to be effective. Since there are competing demands on budgets, and because drugs vary in cost and effectiveness, it is important to be able to compare them so that the best choice of drug is made.

As a group, patients receiving treatment with a drug such as alendronate have an increase in bone density (with a proportion of patients showing bigger increases in bone density than others) and, more importantly, only a proportion will have reduced risk of fractures. Taking prevention of fractures as the aim of treatment, it is known that the most effective way of using such drugs to reduce fractures is to 'target' patients with the lowest bone density.

Economic exercises can be applied to the use of bone densitometry in pre-selecting patients with osteoporosis for treatment. From such exercises it appears that treating patients with lowest bone mineral density and who have had a fracture is a good way of making the most effective use of treatments available. Where a treatment is effective but expensive in relation to established treatments, then doctors can either use the cheaper options or use additional analysis to 'hone down' to those at the greatest risk of fracture to select for treatment.

6.11 What are the drawbacks of such methods?

These models can be only used where there is full information on the costs of treatment and their effectiveness against the three common fractures. Additionally there is insufficient evidence from drug studies to decide on the appropriate duration of treatment for many drugs. Furthermore the effects of drugs on risk of fracture may decline after they are stopped.

There is incomplete information about these topics in certain groups – notably men, ethnic minorities, and other special groups – in whom drug trials have not been carried out. Therefore the main use of such tools has been more or less confined to the major group at risk of fractures, i.e. Caucasian women over 65 years of age.

The prevention and treatment of osteoporosis

7

7.1   What are the goals of osteoporosis prevention?

> The goals of osteoporosis prevention are the maximisation of peak bone mass and reduction of bone loss. Peak bone mass is an important predictor of fracture and therefore from the public health perspective it is important to ensure that peak bone mass is achieved in the population. The principal influences on peak bone mass attainment are genetic.[1] However, the full expression of peak bone mass can be adversely influenced by a number of factors including nutritional influences, physical activity and hormonal status, as well as lifestyle factors such as smoking and alcohol intake. Modifying such factors may increase peak bone mass and reduce the rate of bone loss in later life which is important since the chief burden of fractures is borne by the elderly. Preventative strategies based on public health measures in early life may ultimately impact on fracture rates later in life.

Although risk factors for osteoporosis are established with varying certainty, there is as yet little evidence to show that their modification in the general population has an effect on fracture risk. Because primary care offers the opportunity to provide both health promotion and health care, their role should be to provide such advice to patients throughout life and to combine this with a case finding strategy which highlights those at maximum risk of fracture. In those patients with established low bone mass, modification of lifestyle and allied factors should be considered together with drug interventions.

7.2   How can peak bone mass be maximised in children?

Maximising peak bone mass in children has been explored in a variety of ways, including dietary supplementation and exercise, as outlined below.

CALCIUM

The importance of calcium in determining peak bone mass is contentious. The evidence to date suggests that dietary supplementation of calcium has a small effect on bone density which may be short lived. The brief duration of these effects may reflect a transient effect on the modelling space associated with reduced bone turnover. Although some studies have shown a more prolonged effect, these are exceptional. Thus, whether dietary supplementation of calcium gives rise to long term gains in bone mass still remains uncertain. At present, it is advisable to supplement the diet of children with calcium only if they have low intakes or in those with intolerance to dairy products such as lactose deficiency, coeliac disease or anorexia. *Table 7.1* shows the daily reference nutrient intake of calcium for various groups as recommended by the UK's Department of Health.[2]

VITAMIN D

Although vitamin D deficiency in childhood decreases stature and peak bone mass, its main effect is to induce osteomalacia. The evidence that low peak bone mass attainment in childhood rickets is associated with fracture risk in later life, is lacking.

OTHER DIETARY INFLUENCES

Dietary components other than calcium may be important including high intakes of protein, caffeine and sodium which may cause hypercalciuria. The effects of such factors on fracture risk are however uncertain. Children who consume large amounts of such agents should be encouraged to curtail them or to take additional calcium in the diet.

Attention has been drawn to phosphate-rich drinks which to some extent have replaced milk as the standard fluid intake for children. Such drinks may stimulate parathyroid hormone (PTH) secretion with resultant mobilisation of calcium from the skeleton.

TABLE 7.1 Calcium recommendations based on DOH Committee on medical aspects of food and nutrition policy (COMA)[2]

Calcium recommendations	Reference nutrient intakes* (mg/day)
Adults:	
— men	700
— women	700
Teenagers:	
— boys 11–18	1000
— girls 11–18	800
Children:	
— 1–3 years	350
— 4–6 years	450
— 7–10 years	550
Infants (breastfed only):	
— 0–12 months	525
Pregnancy and lactation	
— pregnant women	700
— breastfeeding women	700 + 550*

*COMA notes that the additional increment may not be necessary with more recent evidence.

EXERCISE

There are several studies to show that exercise in prepubertal girls and pre- and postmenopausal women has a positive effect on bone mass.[3,4] However, the magnitude of the changes is relatively small – up to 3% of bone mineral density (BMD). Furthermore, the effects may be curtailed if subjects resume a sedentary lifestyle. These effects on BMD are largely due to increasing cortical bone cross-sectional area. In adults, increase in overall bone size does not occur with exercise. In children however, increase in bone size may occur especially if exercise is taken during puberty and adolescence.[5–7] Thus, tennis players show an increase in the size of bone and areal bone density in the dominant compared to the non-dominant arm. These short term gains during adolescence may be carried through into adult life.

Most would advise is that regular exercise should be taken throughout life; however, the maximum effect on bone is seen during adolescence. The impact of exercise on bone gain is dependent on the type of exercise. Exercise taken in the form of cycling and swimming has no effect on bone mass. The habit of taking physical exercise during childhood may be important in determining lifelong patterns of behaviour which may carry on into old age.

Taken to extremes, exercise in the peripubertal stage may have an adverse effect on hormonal status in girls with resultant loss of bone stock. Such changes can continue into adult life.[8]

OPTIMAL BODY WEIGHT

Studies have shown correlations between body weight and BMD particularly of the femoral neck in adults. The relationship is a positive one such that patients with a high body mass index (BMI) have a higher BMD and lower risk of fracture. Body mass can be considered as two constituents: lean body weight which reflects body weight without fat, and fat mass. The association of BMD is strongest with lean body mass.[9] Nevertheless, obesity is associated with a relative protective effect for osteoporosis and conversely low body weight in premenopausal women is associated with lower BMD. The fall of oestrogen levels in patients with anorexia is linked with increased risk of fracture. Weight loss accompanied by reduction in fat mass in menstruating women is associated with reduction in plasma oestrone. This is due to reduced conversion of androstendione to oestrone which occurs in adipose tissue.

Many factors can contribute to low body weight in childhood and adolescence including the effects of general medical conditions such as malabsorption or the effects of lifestyle factors including smoking. The relative lack of exercise activity in adolescent girls exposes them to a risk of attaining lower peak bone mass and therefore increased risk of fracture in later life. To some extent this may be offset by the effects of obesity on

BMD. At the other extreme, overexercising associated with amenorrhoea is linked with low BMD.

OTHER FACTORS INFLUENCING BONE DENSITY/BONE MASS

The chief lifestyle factor in this age group, other than exercise, is smoking which contributes to reduction in body weight and fall in circulating oestrone. In addition, there may be an effect by inhibiting osteoblastic activity.

Systemic illnesses of childhood may give rise to reduced sex hormone levels with consequent failure to attain the normal pubertal increase in bone mass, an effect which may be carried through into adult life.

7.3 What non-pharmacological measures can be used to reduce bone loss in men and women?

Investigation of non-pharmacological measures to reduce bone loss include preventative approaches (*Table 7.2*), dietary supplementation with calcium and soy products and the effects of exercise, as described below.

CALCIUM

Although the influence of calcium on the attainment of peak bone density is disputed, there is clear evidence to show that calcium supplementation (in the order of 1 g per day, *see also Appendix 2*) slows the rate of bone loss in postmenopausal women. The effect seems to be predominantly at the

---

TABLE 7.2 Preventative approaches to reduce bone loss (From Royal College of Physicians[10])

Intervention	Bone mineral density	Vertebral fracture	Hip fracture
Exercise	A	B	B
Pharmacological calcium (± vitamin D)	A	B	B
Dietary calcium	B	B	B
Smoking cessation	B	B	B
Reduced alcohol consumption	C	C	B
Oestrogen	A	B	B
Raloxifene	A	A	–
Etidronate	A	–	–
Alendronate	A	–	–

Grading of evidence base: Grade A, meta-analysis of RCTs or from at least one RCT, or from at least one well designed controlled study without randomisation; Grade B, from at least one other type of well designed quasi-experimental study, or from well designed, non-experimental descriptive studies (e.g. comparative studies, correlation studies, case control studies); Grade C, from expert committee reports/opinions and/or clinical experience of authorities.

cancellous rather than cortical site.[11] The impact of this intervention appears more marked in post- rather than perimenopausal women. The effect is chiefly seen in the first year of treatment and seems to be produced by inhibiting PTH levels with a consequent reduction in the number of bone remodelling units. This means that new remodelling units are reduced whilst continued formation of bone occurs at those units already active. This effect can carry over for up to 3 years.

Apart from the influence of pharmacological supplementation by calcium salts, there is some epidemiological evidence that diets rich in calcium (*Table 7.3*) may be associated with reduced risk of osteoporotic fractures. These studies are however bedevilled by differences in lifestyle and other factors influencing the amount of calcium taken in the diet. Studies of fracture incidence show a reduction in the rate of vertebral fractures in those given calcium supplements.[12–14] A combined analysis of these studies (*Fig. 7.1*) showed an overall reduction in fracture risk of 35%. The effect of calcium supplementation on vertebral fracture rates seems greatest when there are prevalent vertebral fractures. Although there is less evidence than for vertebral fractures, there is some evidence to suggest reduction in hip fracture incidence.[15] Thus, calcium alone appears to have an effect in reducing both vertebral and hip fracture rates.

VITAMIN D

Calcium supplementation is commonly given together with vitamin D (*see Appendix 2*). The effect of such treatments in the elderly have been studied

TABLE 7.3 Dietary sources of calcium		
Food	Weight	Calcium content (mg)
Milk		
— whole	8 g	291
— skimmed	8 g	302
Yoghurt, plain/low fat	8 g	250–400
Cheese		
— cheddar	28 g	204
— cottage	4 g	78
Fish		
— sardines	85 g	375
— salmon	85 g	167
Vegetables		
— broccoli	1 cup	136
— carrots	1 cup	50

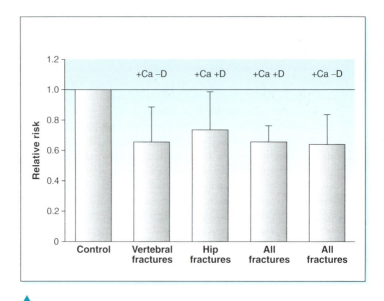

▲

Fig. 7.1 Combined analysis of randomised controlled studies showing the effects of calcium on the relative risk of fracture. A protective effect is evident, irrespective of the concurrent use of vitamin D (+D signifies inclusion of studies using vitamin D). (From Kanis[11])

by Chapuy et al.[16] In this study of residents of French nursing homes, who were given 800 IU vitamin D and 1200 mg of calcium, there was a reduction in hip and non-vertebral fractures. This suggests that calcium and vitamin D supplementation in the frail, elderly, immobile may reduce the risk of fractures. However, another study from Holland failed to show an effect.[17] In this group however the patients were less disabled and community living rather than from residential or nursing homes. Studies from Finland have shown that intramuscular vitamin D (150 000 IU given annually) reduced fracture rates by 25%.[18]

A study from the USA also showed that non-vertebral fracture rate was reduced by over 50% in elderly men and women given 500 mg of calcium and 700 IU of vitamin D.[19]

Vitamin D status is often inadequate in the elderly due to low conversion of vitamin D precursors to vitamin D in the skin (*Box 7.1*). Such rates of conversion are reduced with age and with the reduced exposure to sunlight that occurs particularly in the elderly housebound subject. This combined with less than optimal dietary intake of vitamin D may provoke

---

BOX 7.1 Causes of low vitamin D in the elderly

- Low conversion of 7 dehydrocholecalciferol to vitamin D in the skin (e.g. in the housebound, in dark-skinned races, at extremes of latitude)
- Low intake of vitamin D rich food (mainly fatty fish, dairy products)
- Impaired conversion of 25 (OH) vitamin D to 1,25 dihydroxyvitamin D
- Intestinal resistance to 1,25 dihydroxyvitamin D

---

secondary hyperparathyroidism, itself leading to increased bone turnover and resorption of calcium from bone. It is important to note that the form of supplementation used in the elderly is vitamin D rather than either of its active agents – calciferol or 1-alpha hydroxylated vitamin D. These latter agents confer the risk of hypercalciuria and hypercalcaemia.

Overall the evidence would suggest that calcium and vitamin D supplementation of the diet in the elderly may reduce fractures, particularly in the housebound and less mobile given as a supplement of 400–800 IU per day.

SOY PRODUCTS

Dietary supplementation with soy products has received attention on the basis that those countries with high soy dietary intakes such as Japan have relatively low incidences of osteoporotic fractures. Secondly, soy protein and soy isoflavones have oestrogen-like properties, albeit many times weaker than the equivalent oestrogen 17-beta oestradiol. Evidence for any effect on BMD is at best confined to short term studies of 6 months only. These studies are difficult to interpret because of the variability in dose of the isoflavones used. Lack of standardisation of soy products and the fact that supplements do not undergo the usual trials and postmarketing surveillance of conventional drug therapy, mean that there are no reliable clinical data. Nevertheless, soy supplementation of the diet is very common in Western women and in fact, compliance with dietary supplementation may be greater than that for conventional treatments such as hormone replacement therapy (HRT). Since there is no proven anti-fracture efficacy, such supplements cannot currently be advised.

EXERCISE

Bone mass and fracture risk are linked to levels of physical fitness. Because of this, the effect of exercise has been studied in reducing the risk of osteoporosis in the population (*Box 7.2*). The evidence suggests that weight bearing exercises such as skipping or jumping have an effect on bone

---

BOX 7.2 Beneficial effects of exercise

■ Increase in BMD (especially with high impact, short duration exercise)
■ Increase in muscular strength (reduces the risk of falling, especially in 80+ group)
■ Increased cardiovascular fitness
■ Improved rehabilitation after fracture
■ Improved functional capacity
■ Improved mobility
■ Improved mood
■ Improved urinary urgency

---

density seen in its extremes in the BMD of athletes and in particular those who train by weight lifting. Exercises of short duration and high stress have a trophic effect on bone strength as evidenced by the high BMD of joggers where, in this instance, three times the body weight is transmitted to the skeleton. This compares with the relatively negligible strains put on the skeleton by walking. Weight bearing exercises in which patients use heavier weights and short periods of repetition are more effective than low cycle, lower weight exercise where muscle strength may be increased, but bone density remains unaffected.

The applicability of such observational data to the general population is however contentious. Review of the effects of exercise concluded that there is an overall non-significant effect on BMD, any effect seen being relatively short lived. Since prolonged adherence to an exercise regime is necessary for a sustained effect on bone and because the type and duration of exercise is uncertain, the use of mass exercise programmes to increase population BMD is not advocated.

However, this is not to deny that exercise may influence fracture risk, particularly in the elderly where data from the Study of Osteoporotic Fractures[20] indicate that an increased level of physical fitness is associated with a reduced likelihood of hip fracture. This may be induced partly by an effect on muscle strength and partly by improved balance. Other benefits of exercise in the elderly include improved sense of wellbeing and reduced likelihood of dependency.

Useful increases in bone density in those with low bone density, may be achieved by locally targeted exercise, for example exercises designed to increase bone density of particular sites in the skeleton that are prone to fractures such as the spine or hip.

Where exercise is advised, it is important that the type, duration and frequency are carefully considered, depending on the particular circumstances of the patient. Thus, for children and young fit adults, high loading and frequent exercise such as jogging or other sports may be applicable. In middle-aged, postmenopausal women or middle-aged men, less robust exercise is more appropriate, preferably under the supervision of an expert in the area. Recommendations relating to the types and duration of exercise have been published by the Guidelines Development Group.[21] The particular physical interventions that are appropriate to older people with a high risk of falls have also been published.[22]

ADVERSE INFLUENCES ON BONE MASS

Smoking has several potential adverse effects on bone health. These include induction of an early menopause and reduction in the amount of body fat with consequent reduced production of oestrogen. Loss of body fat may result in reduction in soft tissue cushioning of falls. Low body weight may also increase the risk of fractures. Smoking is often a co-marker of other adverse lifestyle factors on bone such as reduced exercise, alcohol excess and low BMI.

Other negative influences on bone include anticonvulsants, excess supplementation of thyroxine beyond physiological requirements, corticosteroids and other immunosuppressant agents such as ciclosporin and methotrexate. Anti-gonadotrophin treatments (e.g. in the treatment of carcinoma of the breast or prostate) or agents that cause hypogonadism may induce bone loss.

7.4 What drugs can be used in postmenopausal osteoporosis (PMO) to prevent bone loss?

The therapeutic intention in preventative strategies is the maintenance or improvement of bone mass or density. In regulatory terms, prevention means prevention of postmenopausal osteoporosis in patients with osteopenia, whereas treatment is defined as a reduction in fracture risk in osteoporosis (i.e. patients with a T score of less than –2.5 with or without a fracture). In practice, the agents used for both treatment and prevention are the same. The use of preventative treatments should be confined to patients at the highest risk of osteoporosis.

ANTI-RESORPTIVES

The quality of the evidence base for the use of preventative measures for osteoporosis is indicated in *Table 7.4*. The main licensed agents have an effect by reducing the resorption of bone and thus are defined as anti-resorptives. Their efficacy on BMD and fracture prevention is illustrated. It

TABLE 7.4 Treatments approaches in osteoporosis (From Royal College of Physicians[10])

Intervention	Bone mineral density	Vertebral fracture	Hip fracture
Calcium (± vitamin D)	A	A	B
Oestrogen	A	A	B
Alendronate	A	A	A
Etidronate	A	A	B
Calcitonin	A	A	B
Fluoride*	A	A†	–
Anabolic steroids	A	–	B
Calcitriol	A	A†	C

*These agents are not at present licensed in the UK for use in osteoporosis but are used in specialist centres.
†Inconsistent data.
For grading of evidence base, see footnote to *Table 7.2.*

can be seen that the evidence for increase in BMD and fracture efficacy are not necessarily equally strong. Furthermore, the fracture prevention 'profile' of some anti-resorptives is incomplete in the sense that all of the clinically important fractures may not be prevented by some agents.

Studies of drug efficacy in the immediate postmenopausal age group have largely used BMD as the out-turn rather than fracture. The reason for this approach is because such studies would have to be very large and prolonged.

Whilst it seems intuitively logical to presume that an increase in BMD in the postmenopausal age group will be ultimately reflected in later life as fracture reduction, this remains unproven.

BISPHOSPHONATES

The evidence for the efficacy for many of the bisphosphonates and HRT agents is also based on the co-prescription of supplemental calcium and vitamin D. Most of such studies were performed in women with postmenopausal osteoporosis and the results may not necessarily be applicable to other forms of osteoporosis (e.g. in men). However, in practice, anti-resorptive agents seem to have efficacy across different types of osteoporosis.

HORMONE REPLACEMENT THERAPY

This refers to the use of either oestrogen alone or in combination with progestogen (*Box 7.3*). This is usually prescribed in the perimenopausal age

> **BOX 7.3 Types of HRT**
> - ■ Opposed:
>   - — use both oestrogen and progestogen
>   - — if given consecutively – cyclical
>   - — if given continuously – continues combined
> - ■ Unopposed
>   - — oestrogen only

group (*see Appendix 2*). The choice as to whether the agent is oestrogen alone or in combination depends on whether the woman has an intact uterus. Combined oestrogen and progesterone is necessary with an intact uterus since monotherapy with oestrogen increases the risk of endometrial cancer. Progesterone alone appears to have minimal bone preservative effects. HRT preparations come in a range of options and have undergone a continuing series of developments, partly to circumvent difficulties with compliance.

The evidence for HRT in reducing the risk of fractures is extensive but is largely derived from observational data rather than randomised controlled trials (RCTs). The classic study of Lindsay and colleagues[23] of oophorectomised women over a 10 year study period showed that oestrogen reduced the rate of height loss and vertebral fracture rates. A study of the effect of transdermal oestrogen with oral progesterone showed a reduction in the number of vertebral fractures.[24] More recent studies showed a reduction in the incidence of non-vertebral fractures in patients using such treatment over a 4 year period, the risk of fracture being 0.29 compared to 0.47 in patients using vitamin D alone. Where HRT has been used in the secondary prevention of coronary heart disease,[25] anti-fracture efficacy has not been shown.

Despite the relative paucity and the observational nature of much of the data, the use of HRT in the prevention of bone loss and of fractures has, until relatively recently, been commonly advocated as a first choice in the early postmenopausal age group.

7.5   What are the drawbacks of HRT?

Studies have shown that the compliance with HRT is poor – as low as 50% after 3 years. The likelihood of poor compliance increases with the age of the patient. The reasons for lack of compliance are listed in *Table 7.5*. The recurrence of menstruation and the other consequences of oestrogen replacement which can be more correctly thought of as effects rather than the side-effects, are seen by most women as unwanted. To some extent, these drawbacks (e.g. menstruation) can be circumvented by the use of continuous combined preparations or using lower doses of oestrogen.

It is important for women to be fully aware of the potential non-bony beneficial effects of HRT such as those listed in *Table 7.5*. Compliance may be improved by close follow-up by the prescriber or nurse and combined with the use of bone densitometry or possibly bone markers. The chief concern of women is the risk of breast cancer. Although the additional risk of breast cancer above the normal incidence rates is low, many women are put off treatment for this reason. The absolute risk of additional breast cancer cases above the normal incidence rate rises from 2 per 1000 HRT users at 5 years to 12 per 1000 after 15 years[27] (*Table 7.6*). Recent data relating to the Women's Health Initiative (WHI) study[28] which showed increased mortality from breast cancer, coronary heart disease and stroke has also dampened enthusiasm for this treatment. It is of note however that the WHI study was of healthy women rather than women with osteoporosis. The increased mortality due to coronary heart disease occurred in the first year of treatment. This was also observed in the HERS study.[29] There is a small increased risk of ovarian cancer in women who have had a hysterectomy treated with long term use of oestrogen-only HRT.

7.6 How long should patients use HRT?

There is uncertainty as to the appropriate length of treatment for patients taking HRT. Cessation of treatment is followed by a recurrence of the normal rate of bone loss which would have occurred prior to treatment and attenuation of anti-fracture efficacy. Study of women who have had hip fractures shows that the relative risk of those who are current HRT users is 0.35 compared to 0.76 in those who had previously used such treatment.[30]

TABLE 7.5 Side-effects and benefits of hormone replacement therapy

Side-effect	Benefit
Vaginal bleeding	Control of menopausal symptoms:
Breast tenderness	— flushing/sweating
Nausea	— vaginal discharge
Headaches	— reduced libido
Mood swings	— urogenital symptoms
Breast cancer	Fracture reduction
Endometrial cancer	Reduced risk of colorectal cancer
Increased risk of CHD/Strokes	Reduced risk of Alzheimer's disease
Increased risk of ovarian cancer*	

* From Lacey et al.[26]

TABLE 7.6 Summary of possible risks[a] associated with hormone replacement therapy (From Committee on Safety of Medicines[27])

Condition	Age of woman (yr)	Number of cases in 1000 non-HRT users	Extra number of cases in 1000 HRT users over the same period		
			5 years use	10 years use	15 years use
Cumulative cancer risk (ages 50–70)					
Breast cancer	50–69	45	2 (± 1)	6 (± 3)	12 (± 8)
Ovarian cancer[b]	50–69	9	1 (± 1)	3 (± 2)	
			(oestrogen-only HRT)	(oestrogen-only HRT)	
Cardiovascular risks over 5 years					
Stroke	50–59	3	1 (± 1)		
	60–69	11	4 (± 3)		
Venous	50–59	3	4 (± 2)		
thromboembolism	60–69	8	9 (± 5)		
Benefits over 5 years			Reduced number of cases in 1000 HRT users over the same period		
Colorectal cancer	50–59	3	1 (± 1)	2 (± 2)	
	60–69	8	3 (± 2)	5–6 (± 4)	
Fracture of neck	50–59	1–2	0–1 (± 1)	1 (± 1)	
or femur	60–69	7–8	2–3 (± 2)	5 (± 3)	

Numbers are best estimates (± approximate range from 95% confidence intervals).
[a]Risks have been calculated over 20 year or 5 year period per 1000 women with 5 or 10 years of HRT use rather than incidence per 10 000 women *per year* for ease of understanding.
[b]The risks of ovarian cancer with combined HRT are unclear.

Leaving aside the question of the increased rate of breast cancer, these studies would suggest that the length of HRT treatment should be indefinite. However, since prolonged treatment with HRT is associated with a progressively increased risk of breast cancer, reinforced by the WHI findings, the enthusiasm for long term use of HRT is waning. Patients themselves are increasingly well aware of these issues and are likely to have their own views on these topics.

The other complicating factor with HRT relates to the fact that peak usage is in the immediate postmenopausal age group. Given the fact that fracture rates are low at this age, for any increase in bone density to be 'carried through' into later life, when fracture rates are higher, subsequent treatments with other anti-resorptives may be necessary. A contrasting strategy is that anti-resorptives should be maximally targetted at the last few decades of life when fracture risk is greatest. This is supported by health economic analysis (*see Ch. 6*).

In practice, the duration of HRT treatment will be influenced by the factors as discussed, but also by the impact treatment has on the quality of life of the individual woman and her own perceptions of the risks and benefits.

7.7 What preparations of HRT are available?

Given the various preparations and routes of administration, the choices are great. However, at an individual basis choice will depend on the clinical context and in particular the age of the woman. Other factors such as whether or not there is an intact uterus will influence the use of either combined oestrogen–progesterone or single oestrogen preparations alone. Those women with a uterus who do not wish to have recurrent bleeding, may elect for continuous combined treatments or long cycle HRT, or alternatively tibolone. Others may prefer transdermal preparations. The latter have a specific use in patients with malabsorption or liver impairment.

The effective ingredient in HRT as regards osteoporosis treatment is oestrogen, for which there is a dose dependent effect. The minimum effective dose for conjugated equine (o)estrogen (CEE) is 0.625 mg per day and 50 mcg for transdermal oestradiol. At these doses, bone conservation occurs at the lumbar spine; for oral oestradiol the equivalent dose is 1 mg. Those patients who show continued bone loss in the face of the usual preparation may require the dose of oestrogen to be increased.

7.8 Do patients receiving HRT require monitoring?

Most doctors would agree that a baseline pre-treatment assessment is needed (*see Box 7.4*). This should include a full personal and family history, followed by discussion of the implications of the use of HRT or the allied alternatives such as tibolone or raloxifene. Contraindications to the use of HRT as shown in *Box 7.5* will preclude its use. Most information leaflets contain a long list of contraindications derived from use of oral contraceptives where different and more potent oestrogens are used. Most women's apprehensions relate to the risk of breast cancer. Evidence suggests that HRT does not increase the risk of developing breast cancer in the presence of benign breast disease.[31]

A physical examination should be carried out and blood pressure, height and weight measured. A detailed gynaecological examination is not generally necessary except where there is a relevant history. Breast examination is mandatory and if a cervical smear is due then this should be carried out.

Where relevant, other more specific tests may be needed. Dual energy X-ray absorptiometry (DXA) should be carried out in women who are contemplating HRT solely for its bone effects. Where HRT is being prescribed for the management of the postmenopausal syndrome, then DXA scanning is not necessary. Patient counselling should include a full discussion of the potential side-effects and positive effects of HRT.

BOX 7.4   Baseline assessments for patients starting HRT

- History
    - personal history (e.g. thromboembolism, liver disease, breast cancer)
    - family history (e.g. breast cancer, osteoporosis)
- Examination
    - height
    - weight
    - breast examination
- Other tests
    - lipid profile
    - coagulant profile

BOX 7.5   Contraindications to the use of HRT

- Breast cancer
- Endometrial cancer
- Vaginal bleeding of uncertain aetiology
- Otosclerosis
- Severe liver disease
- History of thromboembolism

The maximum drop out rate is seen in the first 3 months of treatment and so it is important for women to be reviewed within that interval. Where vaginal bleeding is persistent after 6 months, then referral to a gynaecologist for transvaginal ultrasound scanning and possible endometrial biopsy or hysteroscopy may be necessary. Given that the major unwanted effects of HRT are largely due to the oestrogen component, it may be appropriate to use a smaller dose at the inception of treatment and to increase this on review. This is particularly appropriate in women who are starting HRT later in life. Continuous combined therapy should not be advised in women who have menstruated within the previous year.

Apart from written information provided by the manufacturers, other information of a more patient friendly nature such as that produced by the National Osteoporosis Society (*see Appendix 1*) are available. Compliance may improve if attention is paid to such details as well as when clear explanations are backed up by written information and women are encouraged to contact the practice nurse or primary care physician/general practitioner supervising treatment.

In addition, the importance of lifestyle factors relating particularly to calcium intake, exercise and smoking should be emphasised, again supplemented by written information.

7.9 What is the role of tibolone in the management of PMO?

 Tibolone is a synthetic compound with weak androgenic, oestrogenic and progestogenic effects. It is effective in controlling vasomotor symptoms and has positive effects on wellbeing and libido. It does not include endometrial proliferation and hence menstruation. The agent causes a significant increase in bone density equivalent to HRT. However, anti-fracture efficacy has not been assessed. Its use should be confined to women who are at least 1 year postmenopausal. Although it has mild lipid lowering effects, its effect on cardiovascular mortality is unknown. Adverse effects include deranged liver function tests and hirsutism (*see Appendix 2*).

7.10 What is the role of raloxifene in the management of PMO?

 Raloxifene is a selective (o)estrogen receptor modulator (SERM) in the same class of agent as tamoxifen. The drug has partly anti-oestrogenic effects and oestrogenic effects in different tissues. Thus it has pro-oestrogenic effect on bone, but anti-oestrogenic effect on breast (*see Appendix 2*). It also appears to have beneficial effects on the lipid profile, although this effect has yet to be translated into improved cardiovascular outcomes. In a 4 year study of cardiovascular events in patients with osteoporosis treated with raloxifene, there was no overall effect on the risk of cardiovascular events. In a subset of women with increased risk however, there was a beneficial effect.[32] However, this study was not designed to evaluate cardiovascular outcome as the primary effect of treatment.

The extent of the beneficial effects of raloxifene on breast cancer is now known.[33] As expected the reduction of breast cancer risk is chiefly seen in oestrogen receptor positive tumours. In the extension of the raloxifene study, the anti-breast cancer effectiveness of raloxifene was still seen 4 years into the study. Overall there was a 72% risk reduction (equivalent to the treatment of 93 osteoporotic women for 4 years to prevent one carcinoma of the breast). The risk of oestrogen receptor positive invasive carcinoma was reduced by 84%. This study found an increase in thromboembolic events compared to placebo. This was equivalent to that seen with HRT.

Raloxifene has no effect on the vasomotor symptoms of the menopause, nor does it have a trophic effect on the urogenital tract. Endometrial stimulation is not seen, therefore vaginal bleeding is not increased.

As regards the effect on bone, raloxifene has been shown to reduce spinal and hip bone loss.[34] A study of postmenopausal women treated with 60 mg of raloxifene found significantly reduced the risk of vertebral fractures. This applied to those with both prevalent or non-prevalent fractures, i.e. 68% reduction in the treatment group in the first year compared to placebo.[35] After 4 years there was a significant reduction in risk of vertebral fractures of 34% in women with vertebral fractures and 49% without fractures. No published data exist relating to effects on non-vertebral fractures.

Raloxifene appears to be most appropriate for older postmenopausal women with risk of vertebral fracture, without vasomotor symptoms, and who are concerned about the risk of breast cancer.

7.11 Which bisphosphonates are used in the prevention and treatment of osteoporosis?

Cyclical etidronate, alendronate and risedronate (*see Appendix 2*) are all licensed in the UK for the prevention and treatment of both postmenopausal and corticosteroid induced osteoporosis. Alendronate is licensed for the treatment of osteoporosis in men. Risedronate is licensed for the treatment of corticosteroid induced osteoporosis in women only, whereas the other two agents are licensed for both men and women.

7.12 How do bisphosphonates work?

All bisphosphonates are analogues of pyrophosphate. Because of the structural similarities with inorganic pyrophosphate, they are rapidly absorbed on to bone surfaces where they are subsequently taken up by osteoclasts. The activity of osteoclasts is inhibited so that bone resorption is suppressed. Formation of bone however is not affected with the result that at the end of each remodelling cycle, there is a net gain of bone. Part of the effect of bisphosphonates may be via their presence on the bone resorbing surface as well as by an inhibitory effect directly on osteoclastic activity. These effects are not confined to bone, and may also reduce the production of ectopic calcification such as that found in disuse (e.g. in paraplegia or after hip surgery).

Bisphosphonates are also used in malignant hypercalcaemia and Paget's disease where their inhibitory effect results in slowing of bone turnover with reduction of calcium loss from bone and relative normalisation of the disrupted bone turnover seen in Paget's disease. They may also have a role in the prevention of fractures due to metastatic disease, particularly breast cancer.

7.13 What is the evidence for their efficacy?

The anti-fracture efficacy of alendronate, etidronate and risedronate is outlined in *Table 7.7*. Evidence of efficacy for each of these drugs is detailed below.

ALENDRONATE

Alendronate is used at a dose of 5 or 10 mg daily for prevention and treatment of osteoporosis respectively. When used for corticosteroid induced osteoporosis, it is also recommended to be taken as 5 mg per day and in postmenopausal women not taking HRT, as 10 mg per day. This has been the most exhaustively studied bisphosphonate to date.

The effects on BMD are relatively large and detectable at both spine and hip sites. These effects are seen in three groups of women: women with normal BMD,[36] women with low BMD[37] and postmenopausal women with previous vertebral fractures.[38]

Efficacy against the clinically relevant fractures was shown in a study of 4432 women with low femoral neck BMD where alendronate was given at 5 mg per day for 2 years and then 10 mg a day for 2 years. Women with a BMD of −2.5T showed a reduction in fracture neck of femur – relative risk (RR) 0.64 (0.5–0.82). The RR of vertebral fractures was 0.56 (0.39–0.80).[39] Another study[40] of 1908 postmenopausal women with BMD of the spine of

TABLE 7.7 Anti-fracture efficacy of bisphosphonates (From Royal College of Physicians[10])

	Spine	Non-vertebral	Hip
Alendronate	A	A	A
Cyclical etidronate	A	B	B
Risedronate	A	A	A

For grading of evidence base, see footnote to *Table 7.2*.

−2T showed a significant reduction in non-vertebral fractures: RR 0.53 (0.3–0.9).

A recent study has shown less frequent dosing with alendronate may be effective, at least in its effects on BMD as daily dosing. Thus, weekly alendronate of 70 mg (35 mg twice a week) and 10 mg daily were compared[41] and showed equal efficacy. Whether there is equivalent anti-fracture efficacy with the weekly preparation compared to the daily preparation is unknown.

ETIDRONATE

Cyclical etidronate is given as 400 mg daily for 2 weeks followed by 500 mg calcium daily for 11 weeks and then repeated in 13 week cycles.

It has been studied in postmenopausal osteoporosis by two RCTs.[42,43] These studies, although methodologically flawed, showed increases in bone mass of the lumbar spine and cessation of bone loss at the hip. A subsequent study has shown a small increase in BMD at the hip.[44] Studies in younger postmenopausal women showed that bone loss at both lumbar spine and hip could be halted by this treatment.[45]

As regards anti-fracture efficacy, both the Storm[42] and the Watts[43] studies showed reduction in vertebral fracture rates. These and other studies show that cyclical etidronate is effective in reducing vertebral fractures in postmenopausal women with multiple prevalent vertebral fractures. Further collateral evidence of the efficacy of cyclical etidronate comes from analysis of the UK's General Practice Research Database (GPRD) which was a study of nearly 8000 age- and sex-matched subjects.[46] This showed reduction in hip fractures by 34% and non-vertebral fractures by 20%: RR for hip fracture 0.66 (0.51–0.85); RR for wrist fracture 0.81 (0.58–1.14). Such evidence and other observational studies thus suggest that cyclical etidronate has general anti-fracture efficacy.

RISEDRONATE

Risedronate is licensed in the UK for the prevention and treatment of osteoporosis in postmenopausal women and corticosteroid induced osteoporosis prevention in women. The recommended dose is 5 mg per day.

There have been two RCTs on the effect of risedronate on osteoporosis in postmenopausal women and both showed anti-fracture efficacy. In one study[47] of 2458 women, treatment with 2.5 or 5 mg risedronate or placebo was studied. The 5 mg arm of the study found a RR of new vertebral fractures of 0.35 (0.19–1.62) after 1 year and 0.59 RR (0.43–0.82) after 3 years. At this stage there was also a reduction of non-vertebral fractures: RR 0.6 (0.39–0.94). Significant increases in BMD at the lumbar spine and femoral neck were also seen (4.3 and 2.8% respectively). In a European study[48] of postmenopausal women with at least two prevalent vertebral fractures, a

5 mg treatment arm found a RR of 0.39 for vertebral fractures (0.22–0.68) after 1 year and 0.51 RR (0.36–0.73) after 3 years. There was also a non-significant decline in non-vertebral fractures. Again, significant increases in BMD at the spine (5.9%) and femoral neck (0.1%) were seen.

The efficacy of risedronate in preventing hip fractures has been studied.[49] This showed that anti-fracture efficacy was confined to women with a T score of −3 who had at least one other additional risk factor for hip fracture. In women with low BMD of the femoral neck, there was a 39% reduction in risk of hip fracture. Those who had both low femoral neck BMD and prevalent vertebral fracture had a reduction of hip fracture of 58%. This study and others like it show that the maximum benefit of this agent is in those with lowest BMD and with prevalent vertebral fractures.

7.14 What are the most important side-effects of bisphosphonates?

Upper gastrointestinal side-effects in the form of non-specific indigestion, at one end of the spectrum, to erosive oesophagitis at the other end, have been described with bisphosphonates. The risk of oesophagitis can be reduced by taking water with the drug and the patient avoiding lying down until after breakfast (*see Appendix 2*). It is particularly important to pay attention to any history of pre-existing oesophageal disorders or other upper gastrointestinal symptoms when considering these treatments. Oesophageal side-effects in clinical practice were not anticipated since the original studies of alendronate did not show this, probably because subjects with a previous history of peptic ulcer or dyspepsia were excluded from these studies. The incidence of such side-effects is likely to be lesser for risedronate.

Using less frequent dosing regimens such as the weekly form of alendronate may increase the tolerability of such agents without an apparent loss of effect on BMD. It is important that patients fully understand not only the correct way of taking treatment in order to reduce the incidence of side-effects, but also to improve their absorption. Absorption of bisphosphonates is poor and is particularly so if taken with food. They should be taken on an empty stomach, ideally 1 hour before a meal and with water only.

Although theoretically there is a possibility of osteomalacia with long term bisphosphonates, in practice this has not been found to be the case.

7.15 What is the relative efficacy of the different bisphosphonates?

There have been no comparative head-to-head studies of the three agents to allow a judgement to be made. In terms of BMD changes however, the phase III studies suggest that alendronate and risedronate have greater effect on BMD than cyclical etidronate. However, the link between anti-fracture efficacy and BMD changes is complex – relatively small increases in BMD may be associated with substantial effects on fracture rates.

As regards speed of action, in terms of fracture reduction, there is some evidence of an earlier effect on vertebral fracture rates for risedronate compared to alendronate.

7.16 How long should treatment last?

The optimum length of treatment is not known. The efficacy studies of the three licensed agents have demonstrated effects within a year which are sustained over several years in terms of both BMD and anti-fracture efficacy. In practice, most would suggest indefinite treatment provided side-effects are not experienced by the patient.

Unlike HRT, the effect of bisphosphonates on BMD appears to be prolonged after treatment has ceased – reflecting the persistent influence of bisphosphonates on bone and their prolonged skeletal half-life. As mentioned (*see Qs 7.13 and 7.14*), it is likely that less frequent dosing or alternative modes of treatment such as the intravenous route may be used in the future.

7.17 Should calcium or vitamin D be co-prescribed with alendronate and risedronate?

Most studies of bisphosphonates have included a placebo group given either calcium supplements or calcium and vitamin D depending on the pre-trial assessment of calcium and vitamin D status. These have also been given to those patients given the test drug. Such supplements themselves may give fracture protection. There is a consensus that where there is inadequate calcium and vitamin D intake then this should be corrected along with the bisphosphonate itself.

7.18 Which patients should be treated with bisphosphonates?

The studies of bisphosphonates have shown that fracture reduction occurs in both the early PMO group and in later ages. However, the maximum efficacy in terms of fracture reduction appears to be in those patients with lowest BMD with prevalent fracture or both. Therefore, such agents should be mainly directed at these groups.

7.19 What place does calcitonin have in the management of osteoporosis?

Calcitonin is a polypeptide produced by the parafollicular cells of the thyroid. It has an inhibitory effect on osteoclastic activity. It also has an analgesic effect, possibly by induction of endomorphins. The inhibition of osteoclastic activity reduces bone turnover leading to increased BMD.

Calcitonin is available as a nasal spray or subcutaneous or intramuscular injection (*see Appendix 2*). In the UK only salcatonin is licensed for the treatment of postmenopausal osteoporosis. The recommended dose is

100 IU by subcutaneous or intramuscular injection daily. The intranasal dose is 200 IU into one nostril daily. Co-administration of calcium and vitamin D is recommended (600 mg and 400 IU respectively).

7.20 What is the evidence for the efficacy of calcitonin?

Studies in postmenopausal women using different doses of intranasal calcitonin have shown small increases in spinal BMD when compared to baseline values. However, no effect was seen at the hip over the 5 years of the study.[50]

Vertebral fractures were reduced by 33% compared to placebo in the group given 200 IU per day. In those women with prevalent vertebral fractures, the reduction was 36%. The reduction in vertebral fractures in the 100 or 400 IU group was not significant from placebo. Although the authors concluded that 200 IU calcitonin significantly reduced the risk of new vertebral fractures, the lack of efficacy in the other two groups detracts from this conclusion. There was no effect on non-vertebral fracture risk.

A review of 14 randomised trials of calcitonin[51] showed that the relative risk of fracture for those receiving calcitonin was 0.43 (0.38–0.5) with an effect at both vertebral and non-vertebral sites. The pooling of data using patients with fracture rather than numbers of fractures resulted in a rather lower risk reduction – RR 0.74 (0.6–0.93) – and the effect on non-vertebral fractures disappeared.

Overall the evidence of calcitonin efficacy in the management of osteoporosis is largely confined to improvement in BMD at the vertebral site and reduction of vertebral fractures. In terms of relative potency, the agent is probably less effective than the bisphosphonates or HRT.

7.21 What is the role of calcitonin in the management of bone pain?

Studies have shown that there is an analgesic effect of calcitonin which may render it of use in the acute management of vertebral fractures. Thus, one study[52] of 56 women showed significant improvement in pain scores over the first 2 days (100 IU subcutaneous calcitonin was administered daily for 2 weeks). Patients taking calcitonin were more mobile and more likely to be able to sit and stand.

These results suggest that the main clinical use of calcitonin is in the management of acute vertebral collapse, where the combination of an anti-resorptive effect, with a central analgesic effect, makes it particularly appropriate.

7.22 What are the side-effects of calcitonin?

The commonest side-effects are nausea, loss of appetite and facial flushing. Allergic reactions are rare. The nasal preparation is associated with fewer side-effects than the parenteral. Long term use of the parenteral agent is associated with the development of antibodies which may reduce its effectiveness.

7.23 What is the role of the metabolites of vitamin D?

Overall the evidence for the active metabolites of vitamin D in PMO is confined to relatively weak effects on BMD and anti-fracture effect mainly seen at the spine. These agents are relatively toxic and there is a risk of hypercalcaemia with their use which should therefore be associated with periodic monitoring of blood calcium levels.

The metabolites of vitamin D include alfacalcidol and calcitriol. The effectiveness of such agents on bone density have been variable and inconsistent, possibly reflecting different states of calcium intake throughout the world.

As regards anti-fracture effects, these have also shown inconsistent results. One of the larger studies by Tilyard and colleagues[53] found fewer fractures after 1 year of therapy; that of Gallagher et al[54] showed reduction in vertebral fracture rates of 45% in the first year. Other studies have shown lack of effectiveness in PMO with prevalent vertebral fractures. Studies from the Far East however have suggested anti-vertebral fracture efficacy. Whether these differences reflect racial or genetic factors or usual calcium intake (Japanese calcium dietary intake is low) is not known.

The chief role of these agents and vitamin D therefore is mainly as an adjunct to more potent agents such as bisphosphonates, HRT or SERMS especially where vitamin D deficiency is present.

7.24 What is the role of anabolic agents in the management of osteoporosis?

These agents include fluoride, testosterone, growth hormone and parathyroid hormone.

FLUORIDE

Fluoride has been used in the management of osteoporosis in Europe for many years. It is however not licensed for use in the UK. The mode of action is thought to be by a stimulatory effect on osteoblastic function.

Although the effect on bone density may be large (up to 40% after 5 years), this is not reflected by equivalent anti-fracture efficacy. In fact, non-vertebral fractures appear more frequently in patients treated with fluoride. The effect on bone density appears to be confined to trabecular rather than cortical bone. The evidence for fluoride anti-fracture efficacy appears confined to vertebral fractures.

In practice the use of fluoride is complicated by uncertainties concerning the appropriate dosing compounded by the high incidence of side-effects which include arthralgia, bone pain and osteomalacia.

TESTOSTERONE AND ANABOLIC AGENTS

Testosterone and the anabolic steroids stanozolol and nandrolone have been shown to increase bone mass chiefly at cortical sites with associated increase in total body calcium. Increases in bone mass in both hypogonadal and eugonadal men have been shown. There has been no prospective RCT of anabolic steroids to test anti-fracture efficacy.

In practice the use of testosterone and similar anabolic agents is limited in application to hypogonadal men with osteoporosis as there are risks of inducing prostatism and prostate cancer with long term use of testosterone. Close supervision of such agents is needed.

GROWTH HORMONE

Growth hormone treatment has been shown to increase bone turnover with increase in urinary bone remodelling markers. However, the effect of growth hormone on bone mineral density is unproven and at present there are no published data on the effect of growth hormone replacement on fracture rates.

SYNTHETIC-RECOMBINANT PARATHYROID HORMONE

Intermittent recombinant parathyroid hormone (PTH) has been shown to increase bone strength and bone mass in animals. Studies in humans have shown a marked increase in bone density with reduced fracture rates.

The anabolic effect of PTH given intermittently is in contrast to the resorptive effect of the agent when given continuously. Study of PTH 1-34 has shown a large decrease in vertebral fractures – 65% in women with low BMD and pre-existing fractures.[55] It has been shown that the increase in BMD after PTH therapy can be maintained and further increased by pursuing anti-resorptive therapy in the form of alendronate.[56]

The application of PTH in clinical practice may be limited by the fact that expensive, self-administered daily subcutaneous injections are required (*see Appendix 2*). There are also concerns about the finding of osteosarcomas in laboratory animals treated with PTH and the risk of hypercalcaemia.

PATIENT QUESTIONS

7.25   Can osteoporosis be prevented?

The risk of developing osteoporosis in later life can be reduced by two approaches: firstly the *maximisation of bone mass in early adult life*; secondly by *reducing the rate of bone loss in later life*. Since the risk of fracture is related to peak bone density achieved in early adult life, measures introduced in childhood designed to increase bone density in the growing and maturing skeleton, combined with interventions to reduce the rate of bone loss in the ageing skeleton, may reduce the risk of fractures in later life.

Reduction in bone loss in adulthood

In later life bone mass declines in both sexes after the middle years of life. To an extent, the loss of bone is a 'normal' event related to declining physical activity with the ageing process. However, the rate and extent of bone loss is increased in those who take inadequate calcium and vitamin D, especially in the very elderly group and in those who take insufficient exercise or expose themselves to other lifestyle risk factors such as smoking.

Dietary recommendations for calcium intake

The UK recommendations for calcium intake are shown in *Table 7.1*. There is a lack of conformity of advice about the appropriate amount of calcium considered necessary in the diet. Despite this, it appears that taking supplemental calcium in the form of 1 g per day may reduce the rate of bone loss in women in their postmenopausal years. Additionally, taking both calcium and vitamin D in later life appears to reduce the risk of hip fractures.

Main dietary sources of calcium

Dairy products are good sources of calcium as well as protein. Some dairy products are supplemented with vitamin D. There is some evidence to suggest that calcium taken as a component of foodstuff (mainly milk) may be better absorbed than when taken as a mineral supplement, i.e. as a tablet. Most Western diets have relatively low contents of calcium.

When correction of low dietary intake of calcium is not possible, then an additional source can be taken. This may be obtained either as an over-the-counter supplement from a pharmacy or health food shop, or may be prescribed by a doctor. Those who have difficulty in swallowing tablets may take calcium in soluble form or as a chewable tablet.

Although toxicity due to taking too many over-the-counter preparations is rare, it is important not to take more than the recommended dose to avoid the risk of kidney stones. Indeed, patients with a history of such stones should discuss this with their doctor prior to commencing such treatments. Occasionally drug interactions may be important such as with the binding of calcium to the antibiotic tetracycline which can result in the reduced absorption of the latter from the gut. Similarly, reduced absorption of iron salts may occur.

Vitamin D supplements

As discussed (*see Q. 7.3*), vitamin D has a major effect on calcium metabolism and a particular effect on the amount of calcium absorbed from the gut and excreted in the urine. Vitamin D is partly manufactured in the skin under the influence of sunlight. As would be expected, the risk of vitamin D deficiency increases the further from the equator people live. Dark skinned races who move to less sunny climates, or in those protected from sunlight by customs of dress, have an increased risk of vitamin D deficiency. Dietary sources of vitamin D are less well absorbed in the older population. Lack of vitamin D contributes to osteoporosis, particularly in the elderly, thus additional vitamin D is recommended.

Dietary sources of vitamin D

These include cod liver oil, oily fish such as sardines, herring, salmon and tuna. Some foodstuffs such as margarine are artificially fortified with vitamin D. The recommended dose for the prevention of deficiency in the elderly is 400–800 IU per day.

7.26 What measures can be used to increase bone mass in early life?

The main influences on peak bone mass are genetic. Thus the *potential* maximal bone mass is 'set' to a great extent by factors which are not currently open to amendment. However, the *actual* bone mass achieved is influenced by a number of lifestyle and dietary factors which between them have an impact on the attainment of bone mass. These include dietary influences such as calcium and vitamin D content of foodstuffs and other dietary factors. Non-dietary influences include the amount of exercise taken, body weight and the effects of illness in childhood. Treatments in childhood including steroids for asthma or chemotherapy for conditions such as leukaemia or childhood cancer may bring on osteoporosis. Other adverse influences on bone mass such as smoking or alcohol excess are sometimes relevant in adolescence. The impetus in early life therefore is to maximise those positive influences on bone mass and to minimise adverse influences on the skeleton.

7.27 Can diet help prevent osteoporosis?

Both calcium and vitamin D are important dietary components in influencing bone mass, as outlined below.

Calcium

Since calcium is the chief mineral in bone (99% of calcium in the body is found in bone), it is important to maintain an adequate intake of calcium throughout life. In practice, most patients with normal diets have adequate amounts of calcium and can compensate for relatively low amounts of calcium in the diet by increased absorption from the gut. Those with low calcium diets may require to take supplemental calcium in the form of medication or may elect to increase the calcium rich components of their diet. It is wise to increase calcium intake during puberty, pregnancy and breastfeeding.

There are widely varying recommendations for calcium intake across countries, American authorities recommending higher calcium supplementation than those in the UK. These differences arise partly because of different interpretations of the body's ability to compensate for low calcium content in the diet. For those who have established osteoporosis the amount of calcium recommended is greater than for the general population.

Vitamin D

Vitamin D has a profound effect on calcium absorption. Dietary sources include dairy products and fish oils. Production of vitamin D in the body occurs in the skin in the presence of ultraviolet light.

In recent years, there has been a decline in the intake of milk in childhood, which is the main source of dietary calcium, especially in girls because of the perceived risks of obesity and the fashion for taking carbonated drinks, which themselves may cause loss of calcium from bones.

7.28   What is the importance of exercise in childhood and in achieving peak bone mass?

Physical activity taken in childhood has an effect on the amount of bone laid down throughout the skeleton. Exercise in children at the time of puberty may have an important and prolonged effect on bone gain which may be carried over into adulthood. The type of exercise is important with emphasis on weight bearing, high impact sports such as running or jogging, these being more likely to increase bone mass than non-weight bearing, low impact activities such as swimming or cycling. Since the amount of exercise taken by children in Western countries is less than in the past – particularly so in girls – there is a need to promote such activities as part of any drive to increase bone health in childhood.

7.29   What is the role of soy supplementation?

Soy products, which are a large ingredient of many Asian diets, have been promoted as a means of improving women's bone health and reducing menopausal symptoms. Populations with soy rich diets have a lower risk of osteoporosis. Soy proteins have very weak oestrogen-like effects. However, the evidence for their influence on bone density is not strong. Most of the studies to date have been too short to be certain of any lasting effect.

A major problem relating to the use of soy products is that the regulation of dietary supplementation is lax. Manufacturers and distributors do not have to prove the effectiveness of such agents by clinical trials. In addition, the components of many of the dietary products sold vary enormously and so comparison between products is difficult. The evidence at present suggests a minimal short term effect on bone density; to date there has been no evidence of anti-fracture effects.

7.30   What is the role of exercise in the prevention of osteoporosis?

Exercise is thought to reduce the rate of bone loss which otherwise occurs in the ageing skeleton. The effect of exercise is not only beneficial to bone but may also improve balance and muscle strength and thereby reduce the risk of falls in the elderly.

7.31   What forms of exercise are best?

Exercise can be taken as weight bearing or non-weight bearing. It is important from the bone health perspective that the exercise if possible is of the weight bearing type. Non-weight bearing exercises such as swimming do not have an effect on bone mass. The most effective form of exercise for increasing bone mass is of high intensity and short duration. However, this may not be appropriate for all ages. It is very important that the type and duration of exercise for individuals is 'tailored' to their physical fitness. Those who are fit may tolerate high impact exercises much better than the less fit person. It is usually advisable to take exercise in a graded/incremental pattern.

7.32   Where can I get advice about exercise?

Your GP may be able to advise you about exercise or alternatively a physiotherapist working in the practice. Exercise prescription schemes in which patients are assessed for exercise are useful where a degree of supervision is needed. Where exercise is intended specifically for fall prevention, then experienced instructors trained in such techniques should be consulted. Other than these exercises, sporting activities in general which combine a competitive element, together with the exercise, may be appropriate in younger and in some older people. Since compliance with exercise regimes is often poor an element of enjoyment may encourage people to continue.

7.33   What other lifestyle factors may be important?

Smoking and excessive alcohol intake may cause osteoporosis. The evidence for an effect of excess alcohol on bone is relatively limited to alcoholics. The advised maximal intake is 3–4 units per day for men and 2–3 units per day for women (1 unit of alcohol is equivalent to half a pint of standard strength beer, one measure of spirits or one glass of wine). There is evidence that alcohol taken in moderation in the form of red wine may in fact have a beneficial effect on bone.

7.34   What drug treatments are available to prevent and treat osteoporosis?

Other than calcium and vitamin D, which are more correctly thought of as dietary supplements rather than drugs, the treatments available include hormone replacement therapy (HRT), drugs with hormone-like actions such as tibolone and raloxifene, bisphosphonates and calcitonin. In men testosterone can be looked upon as the male equivalent of female HRT.

7.35   What are the advantages of HRT?

HRT has beneficial effects on bone mass and reduces the risk of fractures as well as more general effects which make it of most use in early postmenopausal women with menopausal symptoms. HRT is licensed for the prevention and treatment of osteoporosis as well as to reduce the menopausal symptoms that many women suffer in their early fifties. These include hot flushes, sweats, headaches, loss of sex drive and vaginal dryness. These symptoms can be so troublesome that many women use HRT primarily to control such problems rather than for the effect on bone.

   For those women who have had a hysterectomy, the treatment used will contain only the oestrogen component of HRT. For those with an intact uterus, then the replacement therapy will include progestogen. Without this, there is a risk of cancer of the womb.

   Although it had been thought that one of the added benefits of HRT might be a reduction in the risk of hardening of the arteries (atherosclerosis) – and therefore a reduction in the rate of heart attacks, angina and strokes – recent studies have not shown such protection and have in fact shown an increase in risk of these conditions.

7.36   What are the disadvantages of HRT?

Many women do not experience significant side-effects with HRT. However, others find them very troublesome. These include breast swelling and tenderness, recurrent menstruation, weight gain, mood swings and premenstrual tension. Strictly speaking, these effects are more accurately thought of as the normal consequences of taking such agents. This makes them no less welcome to the woman and those who experience such effects are likely to stop treatment unless ways around the side-effects are found. Side-effects are maximal in the first few months of treatment and often subside after this. Sometimes the effects can be minimised by using lower doses at the start of treatment and subsequently increasing the dose. It is important that women starting on HRT for the first time are carefully followed up by their doctor or practice nurse, especially during the first few months of treatment. There is also an increased risk of thromboses (i.e. clots in the vein of the leg) which can be dangerous if these subsequently lodge in the lung as a pulmonary embolism.

   More concerning to most women than the side-effects above is the increased risk of breast cancer. For obvious reasons, this is an emotive topic for many women. The risk of additional breast cancer in women who have had HRT for 5 years is two cases per 1000 women. This risk increases with prolonged use of HRT. Because of this and for other reasons, the length of treatment usually advised is up to 5 years after the normal age of the menopause. As discussed (*see Q. 7.4*), the increased risk of cancer of the womb (endometrial cancer) in women who use oestrogen alone and who have an intact uterus is completely eliminated by prescription of progestogen with oestrogen.

7.37 How can the side-effects of HRT be minimised?

Over many years drug companies have continuously developed these treatments such that many variations are available. There are many different forms of tablet-based treatments of different doses and various formulations of the two main ingredients – oestrogen and progestogen. Usually the two components are given in a cyclical manner, i.e. the oestrogen component given for the first 2 weeks and then the progestogen for the last 2 weeks.

Oestrogen can also be absorbed through the skin applied as a patch. This is a more convenient method for many women. The additional benefit is that the patch treatment is effective over several days. HRT in the form of vaginal creams may be used to reduce vaginal dryness. However, these treatments are probably ineffective in reducing the risk of fractures.

Given all the variations in the treatments available, it is sometimes possible to circumvent side-effects and so make them more acceptable to women.

7.38 Are there circumstances where HRT should not be used?

Women who have had breast or womb cancer should not use HRT. Those women with a family history of breast cancer are also unlikely to wish to use such treatments. It is important for women considering HRT to make themselves familiar with the risks and benefits of HRT by full use of the available literature provided by bodies such as the National Osteoporosis Society or the Amarant Trust (*see Appendix 1*). Where HRT is not tolerated or where patients are unhappy about its use, then alternatives such as tibolone, raloxifene or bisphosphonates may be considered.

 ### 7.39 What are SERMs and how do they help manage osteoporosis?

SERMs are synthetic drugs which mimic some of the effects of oestrogen in the body. Their use in osteoporosis is based on increasing bone density and reducing vertebral fractures. Raloxifene also reduces blood fats and hence may reduce the risk of hardening of the arteries (atherosclerosis).

Because the drug has the opposite effect on breast from oestrogen, its use is associated with a reduced risk of breast cancer. Like HRT there is an increased risk of blood clots, but unlike HRT there is no effect on flushing and sweating, nor does it cause recurrent menstruation.

7.40 What are the bisphosphonates?

The bisphosphonates are drugs which work on bone by stopping the activity of the cells responsible for breaking down bone (osteoclasts). Because they reduce the reabsorption of bone, they are often called anti-resorptives. There are three of these agents currently licensed in the UK: alendronate,

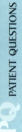

etidronate and risedronate. All are used in the treatment of osteoporosis in postmenopausal women and in corticosteroid induced osteoporosis, although risedronate is licensed for the use of corticosteroid induced osteoporosis in women only. Alendronate is licensed for the treatment of osteoporosis in men.

7.41   What are the advantages of bisphosphonates?

These drugs – unlike HRT – have relatively few side-effects. Their actions seem to be largely confined to bone without stopping other effects which reduce the tolerability of HRT for many women. The evidence of their effectiveness has been studied in much more detail than with HRT and proof of their effectiveness is greater. In addition, there have been prolonged studies in both animals and humans for several years which have shown that the effect on bone continues after stopping treatment.

Continued development of these products has resulted in treatment schedules which may be of greater convenience to patients (e.g. weekly rather than daily dosing) and ultimately less frequent treatments may become available.

 ### 7.42   What are the disadvantages of bisphosphonates?

All bisphosphonates are relatively poorly absorbed from the gut and particularly so if food is present in the stomach. To get round this the three drugs have to be taken between meals. Since they may cause upper or lower gut problems such as heartburn or diarrhoea, it is important that patients are especially careful to take them strictly in accordance with the manufacturer's instructions. Alendronate in particular has been linked to inflammation of the food pipe (oesophagitis) and so it is important that this agent is not used by patients who have abnormalities of swallowing.

7.43   What is calcitonin and when is it used?

Calcitonin is a hormone produced by the body in the thyroid gland. It can be given by injection or inhaled through the nose by nasal spray. The drug cannot be taken by mouth as it is destroyed by acid in the stomach. In the UK the drug is licensed for use by injection into the skin or as a nasal spray and is particularly used in patients who have had spinal fractures, for two reasons:

1. its effectiveness is mainly at the spine
2. the drug has pain killing properties which make it most appropriate to use in such circumstances.

The immobility induced by pain may increase the loss of calcium from the skeleton in these circumstances. Usually after the patient has recovered from the acute pain and is more mobile, doctors may prescribe an alternative to calcitonin to reduce the risk of further fractures, such as a bisphosphonate or SERM.

7.44 What are alfacalcidol and calcitriol and how are they used in osteoporosis?

These compounds are derivatives of vitamin D and are more potent than vitamin D found in the diet. They have specifically been used in conditions of vitamin D deficiency such as in kidney failure, but they are also sometimes used in the treatment of osteoporosis. However, since they are relatively weak in terms of their effect on bone and since they may cause high calcium levels in the blood, they are not extensively used.

7.45 Which other treatments can be used?

Aside from the conventional HRT, bisphosphonates, calcitonin and vitamin D derivatives, there are other more rarely used treatments which include fluoride, testosterone and a hormone derived from the parathyroid gland – parathyroid hormone. These share a common action in bone by which bone is stimulated to produce new bone. Such treatments have the potential to cause greater increases in bone mass than conventional treatments.

Historically, sodium fluoride has been used in Europe, but is not licensed in the UK, except under special supervision. Although bone density does show dramatic increases with the drug, it is relatively toxic and – perversely – increased fracture rates have been found in some patients.

Testosterone is used in the treatment of men with low levels of the hormone and is most relevant where osteoporosis is present. Most recently a synthetic derivative of parathyroid hormone (which is a naturally occurring hormone found in the parathyroid gland in the neck) has been shown to increase bone density and reduce the likelihood of spinal fractures. It is not as yet licensed for use in the UK.

Management of osteoporosis in special groups

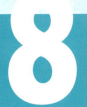

8

8.1 How and where should osteoporosis in men be managed?

> It is important to exclude secondary causes of osteoporosis in men, since the likelihood of uncovering an underlying condition is significantly high. Correction of the causal condition may result in improvement in bone density with reduced risk of fracture. In this regard the most 'fruitful' conditions include hypogonadism, hyperthyroidism, hyperparathyroidism and coeliac disease.
>
> - There are to date relatively few studies of the treatment of idiopathic osteoporosis in men and few randomised controlled trials (RCTs) in which fracture outcome has been studied. However, there are no biological reasons to presume that agents effective in women are not similarly effective in men. The treatment options for men include bisphosphonates, calcium and vitamin D, calcitonin and testosterone.
> - In common with other groups, lifestyle factors may be important to identify. Of particular relevance to men are excess alcohol and smoking.
> - Given the relatively uncertain nature of the treatments for male patients, the high incidence of secondary causes of osteoporosis, and the need for specialised investigations in some men with osteoporosis, it is recommended that most male patients be investigated and managed in specialist centres.

8.2 Which treatments are available?

- *Etidronate and alendronate* – Studies suggest[1,2] that the bisphosphonates, cyclical etidronate and alendronate, both increase bone mineral density (BMD) of the spine and the hip. Interestingly the effect of alendronate on bone density is irrespective of whether the cause of osteoporosis is idiopathic or secondary. Improvement in BMD occurs in men with hypogonadism, treated with alendronate.[3] This study also showed a decrease in vertebral fracture incidence. Examination of the UK General Practice Research Database (GPRD) showed that cyclical etidronate significantly reduces the risk of vertebral but not other fractures in men.[4] Bisphosphonates are the commonest treatment in male osteoporosis.[5]
- *Testosterone replacement* in hypogonadal men increases BMD.[6] The treatment also increases vertebral BMD in eugonadal men. The main concern about the use of testosterone in eugonadal men is the increased risk of prostate cancer that this treatment confers. The effect on cardiovascular outcomes is uncertain, although the effect of

testosterone on cardiovascular risk factors is neutral. Testosterone replacement therapy should not be used in the presence of prostatic hypertrophy. It is important that treatment is monitored by periodic tests of prostate specific antigen (PSA) and liver function.

■ *Calcium and vitamin D* – This combination has an uncertain role in the management of male osteoporosis. Contrasting results have been the feature of studies to date. Thus, one RCT of normal men between 30 and 87 using 1000 mg calcium and 1000 IU vitamin D daily failed to halt bone loss from the spine or forearm.[7] A study of older men living at home however did show a positive effect on bone density and reduction in non-vertebral fractures.[8] A Finnish study also showed that yearly intramuscular injections of vitamin D of 150 000 or 300 000 units[9] also caused a reduction in fractures.

The overall picture is somewhat obscure, but it would seem sensible to consider vitamin D as an option in elderly men, particularly where mobility is poor and risk of falls is great.

■ *Calcitonin* – Overall the evidence for the efficacy of this treatment in osteoporosis is confined to improvement in BMD and reduction in fracture risk at the spine. Men have been included in the published trials and their response to treatment is not likely to be different from women. The main clinical context in which calcitonin may be the treatment of choice is in the management of acute vertebral fractures where the analgesic effect of calcitonin may be a useful adjunct to management. Other treatments sometimes used include anabolic steroids. Recombinant parathyroid hormone has recently been shown to increase BMD at both the hip and spine. However, this treatment is not yet licensed for use in the UK.

8.3 Where should glucocorticoid-induced osteoporosis be managed?

Data from the UK GPRD[10] show that approximately 350 000 patients are at potential risk of fractures due to corticosteroid use. Approximately 161 000 patients per year received corticosteroids for up to 6 months. The commonest indication is treatment of obstructive airways disease (almost 40%). The vast majority of treatments are initiated in general practice. Therefore, the main responsibility for the management of corticosteroid-induced osteoporosis is with primary care.

8.4 What is the risk of osteoporosis and fracture with glucocorticoid use?

Up to 50% of patients on long term steroids have osteoporosis. The risk of fractures increases with the dose used and rises to up to five times control levels for vertebral fractures and two to three times control levels for hip fractures. The increase in risk of fracture with corticosteroid use is detectable even at small doses. Evidence shows that the fracture risk returns to baseline quite rapidly after cessation of steroid use. Overall, the increased fracture risk is about 20% in patients taking less than 5 mg prednisolone; patients taking 20 mg per day have fracture rates about 60% higher than controls.

Patients who use inhaled steroids have a small increase in fracture risk which may be due to the underlying condition itself. Doses of over 700 mcg/day cause significant increases in vertebral and hip fractures. The risk of fracture diminishes once treatment is stopped.[11]

8.5 What therapeutic thresholds for intervention should be used?

A UK Consensus Group[12] suggests that treatment should begin at or below a T score of −1.5 in steroid users. This compares with a threshold of −2.5 T for postmenopausal osteoporosis.

The reason for the lower threshold suggested is related to the fact that fracture risk in corticosteroid treated patients is greater at any given bone density measurement than for non-corticosteroid patients. Part of this increased susceptibility to fractures may be to do with other influences such as the effect of steroid myopathy on the risk of falls.

8.6 How well is glucocorticoid-induced osteoporosis managed in general practice?

The evidence to date shows that the majority of patients do not receive drug treatments even if they have had a fracture. Thus, data from the GPRD show that those most likely to have received treatment are patients who have had a vertebral fracture (44%) compared with only 12.4% of those who have sustained a hip fracture[13] (*Table 8.1*).

8.7 When should treatment start?

Recent guidelines from the RCP[12] advise that patients likely to take oral glucocorticoids for at least 3 months should be considered for preventative

TABLE 8.1 Use of bone active medication in 6 months following a fracture (From Van Staa et al.[13])

	Non-vertebral (%)	Forearm (%)	Hip (%)	Vertebral (%)
Bisphosphonates	4.9	4.4	7.2	33.4
HRT	4.8	5.1	2.0	3.7
Vitamin D	1.8	1.2	3.1	5.3
Calcitonin	0.2	0.1	0.1	1.5

treatment (*Fig. 8.1 and Box 8.1*). Those less than 65 with no previous fragility fractures should have bone mineral density measurements, and the following interventions should be undertaken:

■ Where the T score is –1.5 or lower, then both general measures and treatment should be instigated.

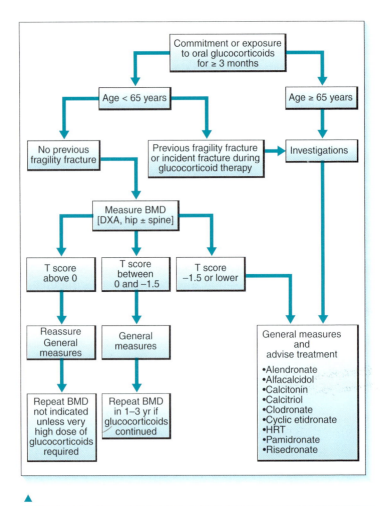

Fig. 8.1 Prevention of glucocorticoid-induced osteoporosis: men and women. L, licensed. (From Royal College of Physicians[12])

> **BOX 8.1   Executive Summary – Royal College of Physicians guidelines on the prevention and treatment of glucocorticoid-induced osteoporosis[12]**
>
> ■ Individuals at high risk should be advised to commence bone protective therapy at the time of starting glucocorticoids, e.g. individuals aged 65 or over, those with a previous fragility fracture (there is no need to confirm bone mass prior to initiation of bone protective therapy in the above patient groups).
> ■ In other subjects receiving oral prednisolone at a daily dose of 5 mg or more, in whom it is intended to continue therapy for at least 6 months, bone mineral density should be considered. A T score of –1.5 or lower may indicate the need for prevention with a bone sparing agent, although the effect of age on fracture probability in an individual should be taken into account when making treatment decisions.

■ In those with a T score of greater than 0, then general measures alone should be advised and repeat bone mineral density carried out if high dose glucocorticoids are required.
■ Patients with T scores of between 0 and –1.5 should have advice about general measures and bone mineral density measurements repeated between 1 to 3 years if steroids are continued.

In patients who are older than 65 and who have had a previous fragility fracture, then the investigations indicated in *Figure 8.1* should be carried out along with the general measures and treatments shown.

8.8   What general measures should be introduced in patients starting on glucocorticoids?

General measures are listed in *Box 8.2*. For obvious reasons it is advisable to minimise the total dose of glucocorticoids by considering steroid sparers

> **BOX 8.2   General measures to reduce bone loss (From Royal College of Physicians[12])**
>
> ■ Reducing the dose of glucocorticoids to a minimum
> ■ Consider alternative formulations, routes of administration and prescription of alternative immunosuppressive agents
> ■ Good nutrition – adequate dietary calcium
> ■ Appropriate physical exercise
> ■ Avoid alcohol and tobacco
> ■ Falls risk assessment in those at risk of falling

such as azathioprine. In the context of obstructive airways disease, inhaled corticosteroids should be the first option rather than the systemic route. Other measures designed to minimise the effect of steroid-induced osteoporosis should encompass not only adequate nutrition in the form of calcium and vitamin D, but also weight bearing exercise, the maintenance of body weight and the avoidance of tobacco and alcohol. In those who have a significant risk of falls, then hip protectors may be provided.

8.9 What investigations should be carried out?

Investigations of patients with previous fragility fracture are outlined in *Box 8.3*. It is important that those patients whom have lost height or become stooped should have an X-ray of the dorsal and lumbar spine. The presence of a baseline fragility fracture increases the risk of further fractures independent of the risk that low BMD itself confers.

8.10 What are the licensed treatments available for glucocorticoid-induced osteoporosis?

These are cyclical etidronate, alendronate 10 mg per day and risedronate 5 mg per day. Although other treatments are widely used in this context, the evidence base for their effectiveness in fracture reduction is restricted to the three bisphosphonates above.

BOX 8.3 Investigations of patients with previous fragility fracture

In patients with previous fragility fracture:
FBC, ESR
Bone and liver function tests (Ca, P, alk phos, albumin, AST/γGT)
Serum creatinine
Serum TSH

If indicated:
Lateral thoracic and lumbar spine X-rays
Serum paraproteins and urine Bence Jones protein
Isotope bone scan
Serum FSH if hormonal status unclear (women)
Serum testosterone, LH and SHBG (men)
Serum 25OHD and PTH
BMD if monitoring required

8.11 What other therapies have been studied?

Table 8.2 outlines the Royal College of Physician's guideline recommendations for therapeutic interventions in the prevention of glucocorticoid-induced osteoporosis.

8.12 How should osteoporosis in children receiving corticosteroids be defined?

There are difficulties in defining osteoporosis in children due partly to the non-applicability of T score methodology in young adults and children.

TABLE 8.2 Royal College of Physician guidelines for therapeutic interventions in prevention of glucocorticoid-induced osteoporosis[12]

Intervention	Spine BMD	Proximal femur BMD	Vertebral fracture
Alendronate	A	A	A[a]
Alfacalcidol	A	A (data inconsistent)	Not adequately assessed
Calcitonin	A (data inconsistent)	A (data inconsistent)	Not adequately assessed
Calcitriol	A (data inconsistent)	A (data inconsistent)	Not adequately assessed
Calcium	Not detected	Not detected	Not adequately assessed
Calcium + vitamin D	A (data inconsistent)	A (data inconsistent)	Not adequately assessed
Clodronate	A	A	Not adequately assessed
Cyclic etidronate	A	A	A[a]
Fluoride	A	Not detected	Not adequately assessed
HRT (incl. tibolone)	A	A	Not adequately assessed
Pamidronate	A	A	Not adequately assessed
PTH	A	A	Not adequately assessed
Raloxifene	No data	No data	No data
Risedronate	A	A	A[a]
Testosterone	A	Not adequately assessed	Not adequately assessed

[a]Not as a primary end point.

(By definition, most young adults and children will have low T scores since they have not as yet achieved peak bone mass.) Differences in pubertal status and body size also complicate the interpretation of BMD results. Children at greatest risk include those with underlying conditions independently linked to osteoporosis or fracture risk, such as juvenile arthritis. Where growth retardation or other signs of secondary Cushing's syndrome are present, then the risk of osteoporosis is greater. The guidelines in *Box 8.2* recommend general preventative measures to be taken as listed. Where treatment is needed, this should be under the supervision of an expert in this area.

8.13 Should prophylactic treatment be given to all patients?

Where treatment with corticosteroids is anticipated to be for 3 months or more, the recommendations of the RCP guidelines should be followed (*see Fig. 8.1*). Difficulties arise however when the dose or duration of treatment is greater than originally anticipated or where short courses of high dose steroids are used.

A pragmatic view is to treat all patients prophylactically at the time of starting steroids. Although the evidence for efficacy of co-prescribed anti-resorptives for patients receiving short courses of oral steroids is lacking, in view of the relatively low toxicity of calcium and vitamin D supplements it is reasonable to co-prescribe them and to use more potent agents in those cases where there are strong risk factors for fracture. For those patients who will require intermittent high dose short courses of corticosteroids, such as those with chronic obstructive pulmonary disease, then it is sensible to check BMD and arrange X-ray of the dorsal and lumbar spine. In the presence of either low BMD or prevalent fracture, or both, then prophylactic anti-resorptive treatment is advisable.

8.14 Should additional calcium and vitamin D be given in glucocorticoid-induced osteoporosis?

Since one of the effects of steroid treatment may be to induce secondary hyperparathyroidism, which in itself causes loss of calcium in the skeleton, most doctors would advise that calcium and vitamin D supplementation is appropriate as a minimum treatment as well as being useful as an adjunct to treatment with other more potent agents such as HRT or bisphosphonates. Calcium alone appears, at best, to slow the rate of bone loss rather than halting it.

8.15 Which treatment should be used for individual patients?

The choice of agent will depend on the individual clinical circumstances, and, in particular, the sex and age of the patient. Thus, postmenopausal women in the first few years after the menopause treated with steroids may wish to consider HRT, tibolone or bisphosphonates. Older postmenopausal women are more likely to select bisphosphonates. Men receiving long term steroids may develop hypogonadism and should be screened for this by serum testosterone, sex hormone binding globulin and the derived free testosterone index. Where hypogonadism is present, testosterone replacement may be appropriate under the supervision of an expert in the area. Otherwise, bisphosphonates remain the mainstay of treatment of glucocorticoid-induced osteoporosis for men.

8.16 How should osteoporosis in children be managed?

As previously mentioned, definition of osteoporosis in children is difficult. The diagnosis should be considered in those who present with low trauma fractures. Where osteoporosis is due to an underlying condition such as coeliac disease or juvenile arthritis, then management of the primary condition may improve bone density. A common complication of systemic conditions of childhood includes delayed puberty which in itself may increase the risk of low BMD, an effect which may be carried over into adulthood.

General measures such as ensuring an adequate calcium and vitamin D intake coupled with minimization of drug effects such as those due to steroids may reduce the risk of osteoporosis. There are no licensed drugs for the treatment or prevention of osteoporosis in childhood. However, bisphosphonates are used in specialist centres including intravenous pamidronate.

8.17 How should osteoporosis associated with anorexia be managed?

Anorexia is associated with risk of low bone mass which may be due to excessive bone loss or, more commonly, failure to achieve peak bone mass.[14–16] The aetiology of osteoporosis in anorexics and in women athletes with amenorrhoea is mainly reduced bone formation which is related to the low body mass index and energy deficit that these patients have. The treatment of both conditions centres on regaining weight and improving nutritional status. The evidence that HRT is effective in these conditions is slight.[14,16,17] Unfortunately most women in these groups are resistant to change of behavioural pattern and the use of drugs. Theoretically, anabolic rather than anti-resorptive agents may be effective in these particular patients.

Since the treatment of established anorexia nervosa with osteoporosis and osteoporosis due to amenorrhoea in athletes is often difficult, emphasis should be placed on preventative strategies to improve eating or exercise habits. Resumption of menstruation is associated usually with improvement in BMD. However, there is evidence of continued 'carry over' of low BMD in women who have had anorexia nervosa of childhood.

8.18 How should osteoporosis of pregnancy be managed?

Osteoporosis in pregnancy has been reported in recent years. It is a very rare complication of a common condition and usually presents in the first pregnancy with vertebral fractures occurring after childbirth. The second form occurs in the last trimester of pregnancy. This usually presents with groin pain, limp or overt hip fracture. Diagnosis may be difficult since bone densitometry or X-ray may not be possible for obvious reasons.

It is important to exclude underlying causes of osteoporosis which may not be apparent prior to the additional physiological stresses that pregnancy places on the skeleton. The increased 'call' on skeletal calcium during pregnancy may tip the balance between underlying undetected osteoporosis and symptomatic osteoporosis. In others, the cause may be more obvious including long term anticonvulsant therapy or heparin or steroid use during pregnancy.

Correction of the underlying condition, where possible, may be followed by improvement in bone density. In the idiopathic group, there are no validated treatments. However, supplemental calcium and vitamin D may be given. These patients should be referred to an expert in the area for further investigation and treatment.

Such patients will require a rehabilitation programme to encourage mobility after recovery from fracture. The likelihood of further fractures in subsequent pregnancies is low, especially when the initial presentation has been a vertebral fracture. Obviously the risk of further fractures in subsequent pregnancy will be related to BMD measurements which should be taken where possible.

 PATIENT QUESTIONS

8.19 How can men with osteoporosis be treated?

Although the burden of osteoporosis falls on women, particularly elderly women, there are significant numbers of men affected by the condition – approximately 1 in 12. Most of the attention of pharmaceutical companies has concentrated on the treatment and prevention of osteoporosis in women. This means that the treatments which are licensed and approved for osteoporosis are nearly all primarily for women. However, there is no reason to believe that the drugs used for women do not work similarly in men. (Obviously this applies to drugs other than hormone replacement therapy, HRT.) However, since the male hormone testosterone is also available, men have an equivalent form of HRT. Studies have shown that the likelihood of finding an underlying cause of osteoporosis – be that a medical condition, such as liver disease, or rheumatoid arthritis or adverse lifestyle factors – is much greater in men than in women. Therefore, it is particularly important for tests to be done to detect underlying causes as well as identifying lifestyle factors which may be contributing to low bone density. Those that apply particularly to men are excess smoking and alcohol consumption. Improvement in lifestyle factors and the management of any underlying conditions in themselves may produce worthwhile increases in bone mineral density and so reduce the risk of fracture.

8.20   Are there any specific drug treatments for men with osteoporosis?

Where drug treatment is contemplated, bisphosphonates such as cyclical etidronate, alendronate and risedronate are the commonest drugs in use. Other treatments include calcium and vitamin D supplements which are often co-prescribed in addition to more potent agents as above. As a sole treatment however, calcium and vitamin D has limited effects on bone and has its main impact in elderly patients with low intake of calcium and vitamin D who may be less exposed to the effects of sunlight on the skin, necessary for the production of vitamin D in the body. This situation is often associated with poor mobility and increased risk of falling. Hip protectors may be of particular relevance in this group.

A specific treatment used in a particular situation is the use of calcitonin in men who have acute spinal fractures. This treatment has two advantages: firstly the drug has a painkilling effect, and secondly the further loss of bone which commonly occurs at the time of enforced immobilisation after a fracture is halted.

Some men develop osteoporosis due to low levels of the male hormone testosterone. This can occur in men who are unwell due to chronic illness, or who are receiving corticosteroids. In this situation, replacement therapy with testosterone – by tablet, injection or patch – may improve bone strength. Some experts have shown that testosterone given to men with normal levels of testosterone may also increase bone density. However, since the long term effects of such treatment is unknown, it is important that the treatment is given under the supervision and guidance of an expert in this area. Testosterone treatment is associated with an increased risk of prostate enlargement and prostatic cancer and other side-effects. Since the chances of underlying causes of osteoporosis in men is greater than in women, and because the treatments are less well founded for men than women, it is advisable that men are assessed by a local expert and their treatment supervised by them.

8.21   What is glucocorticoid-induced osteoporosis and how can it be treated?

Corticosteroids are used in a wide range of conditions including asthma, ulcerative colitis, Crohn's disease, rheumatoid arthritis and diseases of the kidney and lungs. They are used extensively in transplantation surgery in high doses. In these situations the drug has a powerful effect in reducing inflammation and the processes underlying such diseases. It has been known since their first use that there is an increased risk of osteoporosis and fractures. Steroid-induced osteoporosis is one of the commonest causes of osteoporosis and is under-recognised by doctors. Surveys of the use of drugs to prevent osteoporosis have shown that these treatments are not commonly prescribed in either general or hospital practice. Since steroids are often used as an emergency treatment in medicine, it is to some extent understandable that the risk of fracture which occurs often months or years after the initiation of treatment is overlooked. However, it is now so well recognised that the risk of bone loss is great, as is the risk of fractures similarly, that co-prescription of a bone sparing agent should usually be considered.

Bone loss occurs most rapidly at the beginning of steroid treatment. There are three drugs licensed for the treatment of osteoporosis: alendronate, risedronate and cyclical etidronate. The prescribing doctor will usually wish to consider other ways of reducing the risk of osteoporosis including using the minimum dose of steroid possible and will usually advise about lifestyle factors which may contribute to the risk of osteoporosis. These include: inadequate calcium and vitamin D in the diet; or smoking or alcohol excess.

It is important to recognise the presence of major risk factors which may be present before steroid treatment is started, the most important of which is a previous fracture such as that of the spine. An X-ray of the spine may be carried out prior to treatment with steroids being started, particularly where height loss or stooping is a feature. A bone density test may also be carried out.

The choice of treatment will depend on the individual circumstance. For women in their early fifties then HRT may be used, alternatively tibolone. Bisphosphonates are otherwise the main treatment used and particularly so in men. Where low testosterone is found, then supplemental treatment can be considered. Where bone density measurements have been found to be low, then serial repeated measurements may be carried out to assess responses to treatment.

8.22 Can children with osteoporosis be treated?

Although osteoporosis in childhood is uncommon, it is nevertheless important to recognise this and to start treatment where appropriate. There are a range of medical conditions which give rise to osteoporosis either as a consequence of an illness or its treatment. In the latter regard, steroid use is the main culprit, other causes include chemotherapy in the treatment of malignancies of childhood. There is also a rare form of osteoporosis seen in childhood – juvenile osteoporosis, the cause of which is unknown.

In general, the treatment of osteoporosis of childhood is based on general measures such as:

■ advice regarding dietary intake of calcium and vitamin D etc.
■ ensuring that any underlying condition is detected and treated
■ the minimisation of adverse factors such as excessive steroid use.

Drug treatments in childhood have not been properly studied. This area of osteoporosis is obviously very specialised and children should be seen and supervised by an expert in this area.

8.23 Can osteoporosis in anorexia be treated?

Osteoporosis in late childhood and early adulthood is common in two situations: anorexia nervosa, and young women who develop amenorrhoea (loss of periods) as a consequence of overtraining. In both conditions, treatment is based on the correction of low body weight which seems to be the major reason for associated osteoporosis. In each situation, it is often difficult to change the practices which brought on the condition. It appears that drug treatments are relatively ineffective in reducing bone loss or improving bone mass. Furthermore, the bone density of patients with anorexia may remain low later in life even when menstruation has recurred and body weight has been regained. Thus, the emphasis is on prevention by identifying early on the habits which may lead to these conditions. There is a responsibility on sports trainers and teachers who may influence such patients and thus reduce the risk of excess dieting and exercise.

8.24 Can osteoporosis of pregnancy be treated?

This is a very rare complication of pregnancy. The cause(s) are unknown, but some patients may have underlying low bone density for a variety of reasons which only come to light during the stresses and strains of pregnancy. For example, an Asian woman with reduced calcium and vitamin D intake due to dietary and cultural factors may develop the condition during pregnancy as a consequence of the increased stress on the skeleton induced by pregnancy and in particular the effect of loss of calcium from the axial skeleton which occurs during pregnancy. Fortunately, although there is a risk of fractures in subsequent pregnancies, this is not as great as in the first pregnancy. It is important, where possible, to have bone density measurements carried out after pregnancy since this will enable the doctor to gauge the severity of the condition.

The aetiology and management of pain in osteoporosis

9

9.1 What are the causes of pain with vertebral fractures?

The majority of vertebral fractures are 'silent' in the sense of not coming to clinical attention but presenting with insidious loss of height, stoop or as a chronic finding on X-ray. Those that present with an acute fracture usually have very severe pain which may last for several weeks. Chronic bony back pain is common in those who have had more than one vertebral fracture and may have a significant effect in the quality of life of patients. Chronic pain after hip and forearm fractures is unusual, sometimes due to the development of osteoarthritis in the associated hip joint or algodystrophy of the hand.

The cause of the acute pain of a vertebral fracture is essentially due to two mechanisms:

1. Periosteal surfaces adjacent to the fracture site are supplied by pain fibres.
2. The release of inflammatory mediators – including prostaglandin, histamine and interleukins – sensitises nerve fibres so that the pain threshold is lowered.

This combined effect may be amplified by mechanical factors such as nerve entrapment (with associated radicular referred pain), muscular spasm and the effect of bleeding at the fracture site causing periosteal distension.

9.2 What are the causes of chronic pain?

The mechanical factors mentioned above may give rise to chronic pain by the mechanisms described. The emotional component of pain is important, especially where pain is persistent – as with those who have had multiple vertebral fractures. For those who have had their first fracture, the onset of severe pain gives rise to an acute emotional response, similar to a grief reaction. This may ultimately result in withdrawal and depression. The impact of the combined effects of persistent pain in the recovery period with associated postural effects, reduced mobility and function may result in loss in self-esteem and lead to social isolation and withdrawal (*Fig. 9.1*).

9.3 What are the principles of pain management?

In both the acute and chronic state, it is important to identify the physical, emotional and functional consequences of pain. Patients should be given an explanation of the cause of pain and the treatment to be given, the initial emphasis being the immediate control of pain (*Box 9.1*). This is particularly important in the case of vertebral fractures which often require more than simple 'baseline' analgesics such as paracetamol supplemented with codeine. Patients may need further treatments such as anti-inflammatory

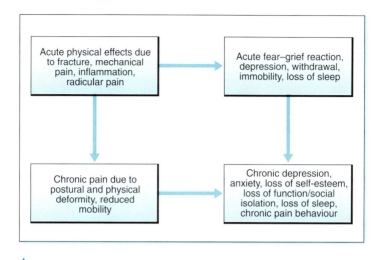

▲

Fig. 9.1 Consequences of chronic pain.

BOX 9.1 Principles of pain management

■ Assessment of physical, emotional and functional aspects
■ Explanation to patient – understandable description of the cause of pain supported by literature and counselling
◙ Pain control:
    — analgesics (simple or compound moving to opioids or non-steroidals if necessary)
    — calcitonin, pamidronate
    — antidepressants
    — transcutaneous nerve stimulation
    — nerve blocks
    — physical treatments (ultrasound, shortwave, hot packs)
    — acupuncture
    — supportive cushioning (NB: avoid spinal orthoses)

---

drugs; however, care must be taken to use a proton pump inhibitor where there are risk factors for peptic ulceration. Most patients with vertebral fractures are over 65 and therefore at risk of peptic ulceration.

It is common to use salcatonin as an analgesic or alternatively – where the patient is managed in hospital – intravenous pamidronate infusions.

Both appear to have analgesic effects, possibly by a central CNS effect and by cytokine inhibition respectively. Salcatonin appears most effective given nasally rather than by the intramuscular route (the usual dose is initially 200 and 100 units daily, respectively). Rehabilitation after salcatonin has been used appears quicker than with conventional treatments.[1–3]

Opiates should be reserved only for patients with intractable, severe pain since the side-effects of constipation and drowsiness may complicate and may ultimately delay rehabilitation.

In the initial stages, most patients are rested in bed with suitable physical support such as a back rest or moulded cushion or bean bag. Local, physical balms such as heat packs or alternatively a transcutaneous nerve stimulation (TNS) machine may supplement pharmacological treatments.

Where radicular pain is a problem, then nerve blocks may help. It is rarely necessary to use orthoses and these are best avoided, since over dependence on them may occur. Anti-depressants are sometimes helpful participating in those with associated disturbed sleep and depression.

9.4 What are the principles of rehabilitation after fracture?

The goals of postfracture management are shown in *Box 9.2*. The pain of a fracture usually settles over a period of 6 weeks (reflecting the normal fracture healing time). Patients who have had multiple vertebral fractures have a high risk of chronic pain, usually on the basis of the compound effects of postural factors due to increased kyphosis with associated muscle strain, radicular pain or pain due to osteoarthritic changes in the spine. The management of such pain often includes continued analgesics and co-

---

BOX 9.2 Rehabilitation after fracture

- Analgesics – co-prescription of opioids
- Tricyclic antidepressants
- Anti-resorptive treatments
- Hydrotherapy
- Graded exercises
- TNS (transcutaneous nerve stimulation) machine
- Postural advice
- Falls assessment
- Home safety assessment
- Correction of falls risk etc.
- Hip protectors, walking aids
- Local group support, osteoporosis educational groups
- Specialised pain services

prescription of anti-depressants (commonly tricyclics) combined with physical approaches designed to increase back strength and mobility. Hydrotherapy is sometimes helpful in enabling patients to exercise in a weightless environment where exercise can be carried out which can increase muscle strength and improve pain control. This can also be of benefit in those patients who have a fear of falling and so improve confidence and wellbeing.[4,5] Initially extension and deep breathing exercises should be tried, moving on to more general exercises including those to increase balance.

Since vertebral fractures are frequently associated with psychosocial complications which may lead to isolation, low self-esteem and fear of further fractures and falls, it is important to assess patients for these factors. In view of the reduced functional status of most patients an occupational therapy assessment is usually necessary in order for patients' full rehabilitation potential to be achieved. In addition, since vertebral fractures predicate the risk of further similar fractures as well as others (notably of the hip), home safety should be reviewed and, where there is a significant risk of falls, appropriate hip protectors advised. Walking aids may also be a useful adjunct to rehabilitation. Risk factors for falls should also be considered. These interventions should go hand in hand with drug treatment to increase bone strength. Bone densitometry should be carried out where clinically relevant.

Inherent in the programme of events is the aim of increasing patients' confidence, gained partly by control of pain and partly by physical and psychological support. This can be supplemented by contact with local support groups (e.g. National Osteoporosis Society – *see Appendix 1*) or attendance at osteoporosis education groups run either in the community or at a local hospital. Where pain control remains inadequate, then referral to specialised pain services may be necessary.

Vertebroplasty offers potential benefits to patients although the exact role of this intervention in the management of vertebral fractures remains uncertain. This method uses bone cement introduced into the body of the vertebra via the pedicles – about 6 ml of methyl methacrylate is injected. This immediately solidifies and so 'braces' the vertebra (*Fig. 9.2*). There are risks associated with the procedure including egression of cement into the spinal canal and embolisation of cement. Kyphoplasty, in which a balloon is inserted into the vertebral body and inflated with cement, is an alternative methodology which again is not yet properly validated.

9.5 What is the role of exercise in the management of patients who have osteoporotic fractures?

The chief evidence for efficacy of exercise is in the elderly where it has been shown to reduce the risk of falls and increase balance, muscle strength and

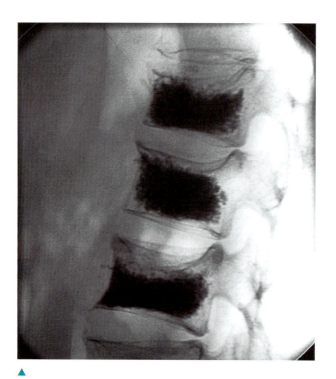

▲

Fig. 9.2 X-ray of upper lumbar vertebrae with bone cement shown.

coordination.[6] Other potential benefits include improved range of movement, aerobic capacity, posture and gait re-education. Pain control and improved psychological wellbeing may also ensue. Since the majority of patients are osteoporotic, and therefore at increased risk of further fractures, the programme of rehabilitation and physical therapy should be cautious and appropriate to the particular individual.

The emphasis is to start with low intensity exercise and low impact loading. Strength training should be gradually introduced. For the reasons described, hydrotherapy may encourage patients to undergo their exercises more confidently than on 'dry land' and may be a convenient 'bridge' between acute and long term management. Increments in the intensity of the programme should be gradual, initially using gravity and body resistance.

9.6   What are the aims of rehabilitation after fracture?

Once patients have recovered from the trauma of a fracture and any surgical intervention, attention should shift towards recuperation and mobilisation. The emphasis is to enable patients to make the most of their potential and so get back to their previous level of physical activity and capabilities. In order to do this, not only is there a need to manage the pain, but also to address the psychological impact of the fracture. For many elderly patients, the first fracture is often 'out of the blue' and is the first herald of osteoporosis. Many are therefore shocked and fearful of exercise and so reduce their chances of regaining mobility and function. It is important therefore that measures are put in place to ensure patients make the best possible progress. Confidence is usually gained by graded physical activity under the guidance of a physiotherapist and with input from an occupational therapist. The former takes a prominent role in the supervision of graded exercises designed to increase muscle strength, mobility and balance – all aspects which may reduce the risk of falls. Additionally, increased mobility and better posture may ensue.

Of particular use in the early management of some patients is hydrotherapy. The weightless environment enables them to exercise free of the fear of falling and so gain confidence. Since some exercises can be potentially dangerous, particularly where low bone density is a feature, it is best to take specific advice from a physiotherapist. Occupational therapists are helpful in assessing the abilities of patients and also home safety. Since most fractures occur in the home, this aspect of patient management is important. Additional help includes the use of walking aids and frames and hip protectors. Some local groups (e.g. the National Osteoporosis Society – *see Apendix 1*) may provide practical support. In addition, attendance at local osteoporosis education groups often under the supervision of a specialist in the local hospital may be of benefit.

Most patients will be prescribed a treatment for osteoporosis by their GP. Where pain control remains poor, then additional treatment such as nerve blocks or other pain controlling procedures can be used. Sometimes it is necessary to refer to a doctor specialising in pain management.

If a fracture has occurred after a fall, then assessment of the reasons for falling is advisable followed by interventions to reduce the risk of further falls.

PATIENT QUESTIONS

9.7 What are the causes of pain following fracture?

The outer surface of bone is covered by a membrane containing within it nerve fibres which transmit the sensation of pain to the spinal cord and hence to the brain. In addition pressure on nerves caused by the fracture may induce 'referred' pain – for instance, pain felt in the lower part of the chest or stomach (e.g. after a spinal fracture). In spinal fractures particularly, and in other fractures to a lesser degree, muscular spasm may in itself cause pain.

The immediate pain after a fracture is due to the pain nerve fibres stimulated at the fracture site. In addition, as a consequence of persistent pain, the body releases chemicals which further sensitise the fracture site.

The emotional consequence of pain manifests itself by fear and apprehension of further fractures in the future. Patients may become withdrawn socially and this may lead to subsequent depression and anxiety.

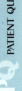

PATIENT QUESTIONS

The aetiology and management of falls

10

PQ PATIENT QUESTIONS

10.1 What is the importance of falls in the aetiology of fractures?

Two of the three common osteoporotic fractures are strongly associated with falls: 90% of hip fractures occur as a consequence of falling, either to the side or backwards; forearm fractures are usually due to a fall on to the outstretched hand.[1] The link is weakest for spinal fractures, but nevertheless, these can occur after slumping into a sitting or flexed position. Although the commonest cause of fractures is a fall, the risk of sustaining a fracture is only about 5%.[1-3] The risk of death following a fall in the UK is shown in *Table 10.1*.[4] As can be seen, the risk is highest following falls on stairs and increases significantly after age 75. The chance of an injury other than a fracture ranges between 40 and 60%.

Fractures after falls occur chiefly in elderly patients with low bone density. In contrast, high trauma fractures in the younger age group are not associated with low bone density.

The incidence of falls rises in the elderly population where the coexistence of osteoporosis is greatest. Thus it is the culmination of two factors – low bone density and increased risk of falling – which make fractures increasingly common in the elderly.

TABLE 10.1 Number of fatal falls in the home per year per million population in those over 65 in the UK, 1995–1997 (From Department of Trade and Industry[4])

	65–74 years	75+ years
Between two levels	2	16
From building	2	4
From ladder	4	3
Same level	3	14
Stairs or steps	21	57
Other	27	198
TOTAL	59	292

10.2 What are the individual determinants of fracture?

These are risk of falling, force of impact, and bone strength. The relationship between them in determining the risk of fracture is shown in *Figure 10.1*. The relative importance of these three factors in any particular patient will differ particularly in regard to age, such that the risk of falling is a stronger determinant of fracture risk than low bone density in the elderly. Conversely, low bone density is a more important risk for fracture in the

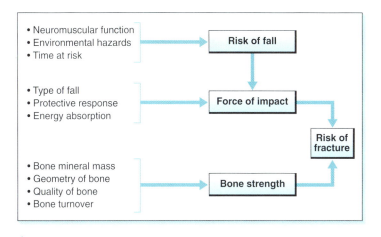

▲

Fig. 10.1 Relationship between risk of fall, force of impact, bone strength and risk of fracture. (After Kannis[5])

younger age group. Although bone density is an important determinant of bone strength, other factors are also important in determining bone fragility including geometrical factors such as hip axis length as well as bone turnover.

10.3 What is the incidence of falls?

The incidence of falls increases with age and is higher in women than in men. The rate of falls in people living at home is between 28 and 35% per annum for those aged 65–74, which increases to between 32 and 42% for those over 75. Residents of nursing homes have the highest risk of falling – up to 80% per annum. A study from Denmark of nursing home residents showed that the number of falls on to the hip compared to all falls was 24% for women and 13% for men. Overall, 36 out of 100 women residents fell on to the hip. The risk of hip fracture after a fall was 0.25% for women and 0.33% for men.[6]

For those living independently, most falls occur during the day. Those in the relatively younger group (less than 75) are more likely to fall out of doors, whereas older community dwellers are most likely to fall in their homes. There is a seasonal variation, with increased risk of falls on cold wintery days. Most falls in the home occur in the bedroom, kitchen or dining room. More men fall out of doors than women – usually in the garden.

10.4 What are the risk factors for falls?

These may be considered as either intrinsic or extrinsic (*Table 10.2*).

TABLE 10.2 Intrinsic and extrinsic risks associated with falls

Risk	Cause
Intrinsic	

Physical and psychological conditions	Decline in musculoskeletal and physical function:
	    decreased muscle bulk and strength
	    increased body sway
	    poor balance
	    poor gait
	    reduced mobility
	Nutritional factors
	Age-related decline in cognitive function:
	    disinhibition
	    confusion
	    behavioural changes
	    poor social integration
	Age-related decline in visual and hearing function
	Low body mass index

Medical conditions	Cerebrovascular:
	    cerebrovascular accident
	    depression
	    dementia
	    parkinsonism
	Cardiovascular:
	    hypotension
	    drop attacks
	    dysrhythmias
	    ischaemic heart disease
	Locomotor:
	    arthritis
	    muscle disease
	Urological:
	    incontinence
	Visual:
	    cataracts
	    other causes of poor vision

Drugs	Anti-depressants Tranquillisers Hypotensive treatments

TABLE 10.2 Intrinsic and extrinsic risks associated with falls— cont'd

Risk	Cause
	Vasodilators
	Diuretics
	Cardiac
	Hypoglycaemics
	Alcohol
Extrinsic	Uneven, slippery surfaces:
	snow
	ice
	Hard surfaces
	Impediments to gait
	Inadequate walking aids
	Unfamiliar surroundings
	Stairs

INTRINSIC FACTORS

Intrinsic factors can be broadly grouped into three main categories: physical and psychological, medical conditions and effects of medication.

■ The first encompasses the *fall in physical fitness* that occurs with age. Muscle bulk and strength and balance decline with age. These changes increase the risk of falls.[6,7] Muscular strength is also related to bone mineral density (BMD).[8,9] For example, grip strength has been shown to relate to femoral neck bone mineral density.[10] Ageing is also associated with a decline in vision and vestibular function. The combination of reduced muscle bulk and power together with reduced balance results in increased body sway, slow pace and poor corrective response to instability and therefore increased likelihood of falling. Exercise may increase muscular strength even in the very old and improve balance and reduce body sway. These changes are independent of any effects on BMD.[11] The general level of physical activity of subjects and their indices of muscle function are related to the risk of falls. Thus increased time in bed (over 4 days per week), increased body sway, Rhombergism, and inability to get up from a chair without using the upper limbs, all predict increased susceptibility to falls or trips.
■ *Nutritional factors* – Low vitamin D intake is associated with risk of osteoporosis and reduced muscle strength and is particularly important in the elderly. Studies have shown that supplementation with vitamin D decreases body sway.[12]

- *Psychological and behavioural factors* – These include age-related decline in cognition and associated disorientation, confusion, or inappropriate behaviour due to disinhibition which may bring with them a reduced appreciation of the risks of falling. Behavioural patterns predicate the risks of falls including self-neglect and poor social integration into the community.
- *Medical conditions* – Many medical conditions are associated with the risk of falls, including cerebrovascular disease, for example transient ischaemic attacks (TIAs), cerebrovascular accidents (CVAs) and vertebrobasilar insufficiency or other causes of drop attacks including dysrhythmias. Reduced visual acuity is common in the elderly, usually due to either cataracts or macular degeneration. Rheumatic complaints with associated arthritis of major weight bearing joints or those associated with foot conditions are of increasing importance in the elderly. Other common risk factors include incontinence or urinary frequency.
- *Effects of medication* – Medications associated with increased liability to falls include hypnotics, hypotensive treatments, diuretics and cardiac medication. High alcohol intake is also an important factor, particularly in the context of elderly, frail men, living alone who are often socially isolated and coexistently physically neglected.

EXTRINSIC FACTORS

Extrinsic factors relate to the environmental context likely to lead to falls, for example:

- *Uneven or slippery surfaces* – These are commonly due to snow or ice, or uneven surfaces due to misfitting carpets.
- *Stairs* – Stairs are implicated in at least 10% of deaths related to falls.

There are a large number of causes for falls. These have been reviewed[13] from published data and the most important ones identified are shown in *Table 10.3.*

10.5 When are people at greatest risk of falling?

Characteristically the risk of falling in the elderly is maximal at the time of ill-health which commonly results in a combination of disorientation and behavioural changes. This may occur for example when patients are admitted to hospital with intercurrent illnesses or when transferred to nursing homes. The liability to fall is maximal, in the latter context, within the first few weeks of admission. Less elderly people (i.e. those aged 65–74) who fall, characteristically do so out of doors and usually in winter.

TABLE 10.3 Summary of 12 major studies of causes of falls (Modified from Masud[13])

Cause	Percentage
Accident/environment	31
Gait/balance/weakness	17
Dizziness/vertigo	13
Drop attacks	9
Confusion	5
Postural hypotension	3
Visual disorder	2
Syncope	0.3
Other	15

10.6 Can the risk of falls be reduced?

A study of patients who presented to a UK Accident and Emergency Department because of falling showed that interventions designed to assess medical reasons for fall, combined with an occupational therapy assessment resulted in prolonged reduction in the risk of further falls.[14] Other studies from the USA have also shown that fall frequency can be reduced when medications are reviewed and balance and gait training introduced.[15] However, the incidence of fractures was not reduced. Other studies have shown that exercise regimes can reduce risk of falls in the community.

The role of improving home safety is uncertain. It appears that correction of home hazards, although important, probably needs to be linked with review of medical conditions and drug treatments in order to be effective in reducing the risk of falling.

10.7 What interventions can be employed?

Interventions should follow from an understanding of the cause of falls.

Improvement in the physical and psychological wellbeing of patients is at the heart of management. Essentially this means adopting means to increase physical fitness and an assessment of any psychological contributing factors, together with improvement in social integration and with support from care agencies where necessary. This should be combined with general health measures including correction of vitamin D deficiency and the use of treatments for osteoporosis. Where medical conditions are thought to be important, their improvement may reduce the risk of further falls (e.g. treating heart failure, parkinsonism, hypotension, etc.).

Medical assessment should include a review of vision and lower body strength – this is simply assessed by asking the patient to stand unaided from a chair. Where poor muscle strength or balance is found, then formal assessment should be undertaken by a physiotherapist along with advice on specific exercises to suit the individual.

Weight bearing exercises in the form of walking for 30 minutes at least three times a week is commonly advised. More specific exercise and balance training may reduce the risk of instability. Walking aids may improve mobility and safety.

Hip protectors have been shown to reduce the risk of hip fractures by 56% per year.[16] They act by absorbing energy at the site of impact. Women with hip fractures are likely to be underweight compared with controls and susceptibility to fracture is partly explained by reduced soft tissue covering the trochanter and buttocks. Widespread use of hip protectors is limited because of poor compliance. Only about 50% of subjects use them, partly due to discomfort and the compounding effect of other factors such as continence problems, difficulty in putting them on, or forgetfulness.

Although as discussed, the evidence that improving home safety per se does not reduce the risk of falls, on an individual basis, it is sensible to assess home circumstances and to make adjustments as necessary. Some of the possible measures are indicated in *Table 10.4*.

10.8 What guidelines for fall prevention are available?

Guidelines for the prevention of falls in older people have been published.[17] The National Service Framework for Older People (as applicable to England and Wales, with Scottish and Welsh variations) includes falls as one of the standards (Standard 6).[18] This has been given added impetus by the suggested timetable for falls services to be set up. The National Osteoporosis Society publication *Primary Care Strategy for Osteoporosis and Falls* is also an additional and valuable resource for those working in primary care.[19]

TABLE 10.4 Interventions after falls

Measures to reduce the risk of falls	Home safety measures

Improvement in physical strength:
  exercises
  walking
  balance training
	Good lighting, long life bulbs, etc.
	Letter box cage
	Avoid clutter
	Avoid loose carpets

Use of vitamin D & calcium	Use of flat-soled shoes
Review of medical conditions associated with falls	Avoid going out in wet, snow or ice
Review of medications	Grab rails for stairs, toilet, shower
Use of hip protectors and walking aids	Telephone by the bed Use of commode by the bed Alarm system

PQ PATIENT QUESTIONS

10.9 If I have osteoporosis, does this mean that my bones will break if I fall over?

Wrist and hip fractures commonly occur after a fall. Falls may cause high stresses to be applied to bones. Where osteoporosis is present, then the risk of fracture is greater. Most patients with osteoporotic bones do not usually sustain fractures in the course of everyday life. However, the force applied to a weakened bone by a fall is sufficient to result in fracture. The commonest type of fall is on to the outstretched hand which often occurs in icy or slippery circumstances. Older men and women tend to fall to the side and are at risk of hip fracture. This happens because the weight of the body impacts on to the hip as the outer bony part of the hip strikes the pavement or floor. The direct force applied at this site is in excess of the bony strength. Spinal fractures are only exceptionally caused by falls. These can however occur after twisting or jolting movements of the spine.

In summary therefore, two 'ingredients' come together to produce a fracture: low bone strength due to osteoporosis; and injury or trauma, commonly a fall.

10.10 Which people are most prone to falling?

The risk of falling increases with age in both men and women. The risk is greater for women than men at any age but particularly so after middle age. The risk of falling is greatest for those in residential or nursing homes.

The causes of falls are numerous. They include the effects of reduced muscle strength, decline in mobility and decreased responsiveness to instability (i.e. an inability to react to the fall). Declining eyesight and balance – common consequences of ageing – also exacerbate the problem. In addition, medical conditions themselves increase the risk of falling by differing effects. These include poor mobility due to arthritis, weakness due to strokes or sudden loss of consciousness which can occur in those patients subject to 'drop' attacks – due to irregularity of the heart beat or small strokes (transient ischaemic attacks – TIAs). Disorientation and confusion which may occur after an acute illness such as pneumonia also increase the risk of falling. Other risk factors include the effects of drugs, for example blood pressure-lowering agents which may cause dizziness, drugs which may affect the heart beat, sedatives or allied drugs which may induce drowsiness. Most falls occur in the home due to hazards such as loose rugs, poor lighting or slippery surfaces.

10.11 How can falls be prevented?

The more active and generally fit a person is in older life, the less likelihood there is of falling. Therefore, regular exercise is advisable for the general population throughout life. It is also known that a good diet with adequate calcium and vitamin D is needed to reduce the risk of fractures in the elderly. The kind of exercise advised will depend on the fitness of the individual. However, regular weight bearing exercise in the form of walking at least three times per week for 30 minutes is usually suggested since ill-health contributes to the risk of falling.

Attention to the underlying cause may reduce the risk of falling. Falls often occur when people are getting up from a chair or negotiating stairs. If dizziness occurs when getting up, then preventative action such as getting up slowly or using a grab rail may help. Review of medications should be undertaken to see if side-effects have contributed to the fall. Where a fall has occurred in the domestic setting, then a home assessment by an occupational therapist may identify dangerous practices which can then be addressed. In some circumstances, the doctor or therapist may advise the use of padded hip protectors or walking aids such as a walking stick or walking frame.

10.12   What are hip protectors?

These are padded underwear given to patients with a risk of falling. They reduce the risk of a fracture by absorbing the energy of the fall into the polypropylene padding overlying the bony outer part of the hip.

Future developments

11

11.1 What are the likely future developments in the definition and diagnosis of osteoporosis?

The World Health Organization (WHO) definition of osteoporosis incorporates within it both bone mass or density reduction with a qualitative deterioration in bone. A recent redefinition of osteoporosis is as a skeletal disorder characterised by compromised bone strength, predisposing a person to an increased risk of fracture.[1] In practice, measurement of bone mineral density (BMD) is used for definition purposes.

■ *Bone mineral density, age and fracture* – BMD, age and prevalent fracture are the most important predictors of fracture. There is an overlap between BMD measurements of patients with and those without fractures. Leaving aside other factors which may give rise to this lack of discrimination – such as propensity to fall – part of the lack of a clear-cut dissociation between the two groups may be to do with bone quality. Future methods may be adopted to address this component of the definition.

■ *Ultrasound* – To date, ultrasound techniques have not been fully validated. However, like DXA they are useful tools to predict fracture. Other methods developed from MRI and the application of fractal analysis to digitised X-rays may be applicable in the research or specialist bone centre setting. However, they are unlikely to become generally available. The portability, cheapness and relative simplicity of use of ultrasound-based techniques together with their usefulness in fracture predictability means that such systems are likely to be taken up increasingly in general practice.

■ *Epidemiology* – The usefulness of bone mineral density as a predictor of fracture lies in the strength of epidemiological data to support this association. Most of the evidence in this field relates to female Caucasians with relatively scant data for other ethnic groups and men. Therefore epidemiological data of this nature are needed to enable a fuller understanding of the risk of fracture in such groups. The applicability of the WHO definition for men and these other groups will also need to be established.

■ *Site of measurement/fracture assessment database* – As regards the optimum site for measurement of BMD and the relevant database to use for fracture assessment, the hip is the most important fracture and since the USA's National Health and Nutrition Examination Survey (NHANES) database is well validated, it is likely that in future measurements of total hip rather than femoral neck will be adopted as the preferred site of measurement. In those under 65 this will usually be combined with an axial measurement carried out at the spine.

Those over this age will have a peripheral site measurement of which the os calcis or alternatively, the forearm appear to be the most appropriate.

11.2 How will fracture management change in the future?

Although fractures are the clinical consequence of osteoporosis, it is common for patients with wrist or vertebral fractures to go untreated both in primary and secondary care. Systems to highlight these fractures will be set up in secondary care (e.g. fracture liaison services). By the same token, it is likely that at the other end of the range of expression of osteoporosis (i.e. hip fractures in the elderly), services will develop to provide a means for guiding such patients to treatment and interventions to reduce the risk of falls. Vertebral fractures are a strong predictor for further fractures at this site, as well as at the hip. They are however under-recognised. It is appropriate therefore to screen for vertebral fractures at the time of BMD measurement using either simple X-ray of the spine or vertebral morphometry such as individual vertebral assessment which applies lateral morphometry to the spine at the time of bone density measurement.

11.3 Will the focus of case finding change?

Since the risk of first fracture is less than 3% over the first 5 years after the menopause and does not rise significantly until age 70, it is logical to shift the focus of case finding to women in their late sixties, using the strong risk factors identified in the Royal College of Physician Guidelines[2] and those derived from the Study of Osteoporotic Fractures,[3] to highlight those at greatest risk. The justification of such a policy will ultimately hinge on the costs of tests and treatments, weighed against the benefit of such an approach in fractures prevented: in short, the health economic implications of this policy.

11.4 Is the T scoring system here to stay?

Whilst the T score system has been generally adopted, it does bring with it significant disadvantages including variability of results across different sites within the skeleton and the fact that it cannot be applied between different methodologies (e.g. bone densitometry, ultrasound). The strength of fracture risk predictability varies between sites, and T score measurements at different ages imply different risks of fracture; for example, a T score of −2.5 in a 50-year-old woman is associated with a lower risk of fracture than at age 80. Therefore, it is likely that transformation of T score measurements into absolute risk of fracture will be the future model by which BMD measurements are interpreted. The T score systems will still be used to establish the diagnosis.

The use of absolute risk assessment will enable the physician and patient to decide on drug therapy. Such risk assessment is best represented in terms of short term absolute risks over a 5–10 year period. In practice, the application of this methodology will be dependent on the data relating to fracture incidence supporting such databases. Thresholds for particular interventions will be 'set' such that where the risk of fracture is highest, then the most effective treatments will be directed. With the advent of highly effective and expensive treatments such as parathyroid hormone (PTH), this will be used as a means of directing treatments most effectively.

Such models may ultimately incorporate the results of biochemical markers of bone turnover which are independent predictors of risk fracture and bone loss. However, the strength of association and the exact role of bone markers in fracture prediction are uncertain and these, combined with the difficulties relating to the standardisation of such tests, make their future use uncertain.

11.5 Is it likely that HRT will continue to be widely used to treat osteoporosis, given recent developments?

Turning to the likely trends in the management of postmenopausal osteoporosis, it is clear that, for a variety of reasons, HRT is likely to have a reducing role. The main reasons have been discussed (*see Ch. 6*) and include concerns about breast cancer risk and increased risk of coronary heart disease (CHD). Although the absolute risk of cancer is low, because of patients' perceived risk and the most recent information relating to CHD risk, problems of long term compliance and uncertainty about the appropriate length of treatment as well as the attenuation of anti-fracture efficacy after cessation of therapy and other concerns (e.g. ovarian cancer risk), decline in the use of HRT is likely. In addition, the advantages of other treatments also mean that these will feature higher in the order of treatment options than before. Leaving aside the question of the anti-fracture efficacy profiles of some agents which are incomplete (e.g. complete lack of anti-fracture efficacy for tibolone), it is probable that there will be an increase in the use of agents such as raloxifene, tibolone and the major bisphosphonates, risedronate and alendronate.

11.6 What other therapies are likely to be used in place of HRT?

Since raloxifene has anti-cancer efficacy, and notwithstanding the fact that this is not a licensed indication for its use, in practice it is likely that it may have a significant increased use. However, anti-fracture efficacy at the hip has not yet been demonstrated.

Bisphosphonates, like HRT before them are becoming 'repackaged', such that different methods of administration – daily, weekly and monthly treatment regimens – will be developed. It is important that anti-fracture efficacy be established for these different regimens. Studies suggest that anti-fracture effectiveness is maintained, at least in the case of alendronate where prolonged treatment up to 10 years has been studied. This evidence also suggests that those who stop treatment after 5 years appear to maintain their bone mineral density with no increase in bone loss. Bone marker turnover studies revert to premenopausal rates, i.e. there is no evidence for an acceleration of bone loss after cessation of therapy. This early evidence suggests that prolonged treatment with bisphosphonates has continued anti-fracture efficacy. If such findings are common to other drugs of this class, then this may lead to their extensive and long term use.

Further developments of the selective (o)estrogen receptor modulator (SERM) concept are likely to be followed by treatments having oestrogenic effects on central nervous, cardiovascular and genitourinary systems and on the skin, and antagonistic effects on the uterus and breast.

Increase in the use of anabolic agents such as PTH is likely. Their advantage lies in their stimulatory effect on bone formation, rather than inhibitory effect on bone destruction, resulting in potentially greater increases in bone mineral density and more importantly anti-fracture efficacy than with anti-resorptives. It has to be remembered that the link between BMD and anti-fracture efficacy is not necessarily straightforward as evidenced by the use of fluoride in the past. In this situation, impressive increases in BMD are not matched by equivalent anti-fracture efficacy and in fact, overall fracture incidence may be reduced. Cost utility analysis may direct interventions to the most appropriate groups. Despite the apparent attractiveness of PTH, the fact that it is given by parenteral route, its expense and lack of long term data mean that its use will be relatively limited to special groups.

11.7 What about combined treatments?

The advent of combined treatments (e.g. PTH and oestrogen) or variations such as intermittent PTH followed by a bisphosphonate are likely. The development of such regimens will need validation to ensure that fracture prevention is better than with single agents. Combinations of agents which are of the same class of action (e.g. anti-resorptives) may have less effect on BMD than combined or cyclical anabolic and anti-resorptive agents. The combination of HRT and alendronate has shown significant increases in BMD. As indicated, such combinations are likely to be reserved for patients with the most difficult conditions (e.g. those who have not responded to conventional treatments). There are of course risks attached to the strategy, not least those of increased expense and risk of side-effects. Additionally as yet, anti-fracture efficacy data are not available.

11.8 Which factors may increase patient compliance in the future?

Methods to increase compliance will be important to pursue for obvious reasons. This is an important topic, particularly where long term treatment of a condition with a delayed ultimate manifestation such as osteoporosis is considered. Although compliance with HRT is known to be poor, the compliance issue is also important for bisphosphonates. This is particularly the case for older patients who may have difficulty in adhering to the correct method and timing of taking these drugs. Apart from the 'repackaging' of bisphosphonates by different treatment schedules including the intravenous route, other means such as the regular review of patients on treatment, use of bone markers or BMD, are likely to be used to increase compliance. Regular surveillance of patients on treatment should include simple measurements such as height or X-ray of the spine where significant height loss has occurred or alternatively the use of vertebral morphometry combined with BMD measurements.

11.9 How may the risks of falls be reduced in the future?

Turning to the question of reduction of falls, evidence for reduction of fractures following fall prevention strategies is not currently apparent. Interventions to reduce the risk of falls have relied on the combination of modification of the various factors responsible for falls, both intrinsic to the patient (e.g. correction of visual handicap, poor stability) and extrinsic (factors to do with the environment). Because of the non-standard nature of studies in this area, the importance of the components of such interventions is uncertain. At present the major impact of any fall prevention programmes seems to be related to effects on exercise and balance. The role of fall prevention strategies either to the population as a whole or targeted to fallers is uncertain. It is likely that most attention in the future will be directed to those at high risk of falls rather than a population-based approach

On the related issue of exercise advice to the population or individual, evidence would suggest that the best impact on bone mineral density is chiefly seen in the adolescent and older groups. Exercise is associated with a reduced risk of falls, and better balance and muscle strength. However, for interventions based on exercises to be effective, continued lifelong maintenance of exercise is required. Compliance with exercise regimes is poor. Greater attention to promoting bone health in childhood and later life should be the priority of those responsible for public health. Other interventions should include the widespread use of calcium and vitamin D, the latter given as annual doses, depending on the results of trials in this area.

Although hip protectors have been shown to be effective when worn, poor compliance limits their usefulness. Alternative methods will need to be developed to improve compliance.

11.10 Which main group of people should be systematically assessed for risk of fracture?

Since the 'richest seam' of hip fractures is found in residential and nursing homes, systems and practices to identify those at risk will need to be used to ensure that risk of fracture is assessed and interventions followed, such as review of drug use, assessment of fall risk, assessment of mobility and stability, and use of lower beds and cushioned floors. Such good practice should be the subject of review, for example by publication of nursing home standards with regular audit of numbers of falls and their consequences. These initiatives are in step with the UK's National Service Framework for Older People[4] which suggests audit of local services and the initiation of interventions to reduce the incidence of falls.

APPENDIX 1
Useful addresses and websites for the GP and the patient

NATIONAL SOCIETIES

National Osteoporosis Society
Camerton
Bath
BA2 0PJ
UK
Tel.: (+44) (0)1761 471771
Fax: (+44) (0)1761 471104
Professional Helpline: (+44) (0)1761 472721
Email: info@nos.org.uk
Website: http://www.nos.org.uk

Primary Care Rheumatology Society
55 South Parade
Northallerton
North Yorkshire
DL7 8SL
UK

International Osteoporosis Foundation (IOF)
71 Cours Albert Thomas
69447
Lyon
Cedex 03
France
Website: http://www.osteofound.org

National Osteoporosis Foundation (USA)
1232, 22nd Street NW
Washington
DC 20037-1292
USA
Tel.: (+1) 202 223 2226
Fax: (+1) 202 223 2237
Website: http://www.nof.org

International Bone and Mineral Society (IBMS)
2025 M Street NW – Suite 800
Washington
DC 20036-3309
USA
Tel.: (+1) 202 367 1121
Fax: (+1) 202 367 2121
Website: http://www.osteo.org/links.html

OTHER EDUCATIONAL RESOURCES

■ *University of Washington – Osteoporosis and Bone Physiology*: information relating to osteoporosis and allied metabolic diseases – http://courses.washington.edu/bonephys

■ *Advances in osteoporosis:* electronic journal containing abstracts and critical analysis of world literature – http://www.bonekey-ibms.org

■ *Doctor's Guide – Osteoporosis*: information resources for professionals and patients including medical news, drug information, discussion groups – http://www.pslgroup.com/OSTEOPOROSIS.htm

■ *Essential Facts*: information sheets including those on osteoporosis written for patients by GPs – http://www.healthinfocus.co.uk

■ *NetDoctor*: patient information site offering interactive forum – http://www.netdoctor.co.uk

■ *PRAXIS*: American patient and doctor reference source providing practical answers for patients and doctors – http://www.praxis.md

OTHER PROFESSIONAL EDUCATIONAL RESOURCES

■ *American Society for Bone and Mineral Research*: professional, medical and scientific society incorporating clinical and experimental scientists. Physicians involved in the study of bone and mineral metabolism – http://www.asbmr.org

■ *Bone and Joint Decade*: the goal of the Bone and Joint Decade is to improve the health related quality of life for people with musculoskeletal disorders, increasing awareness and promoting positive actions to combat the suffering and costs associated with such disorders including osteoporosis – http://www.boneandjointdecade.org

■ *Bone and Tooth Society*: premier scientific society for clinicians and scientists involved in medical management and research of bone disease – http://www.batsoc.org.uk

■ *British Medical Association*: doctors' professional society incorporating scientific functions and the production of major journals – http://www.bma.org.uk

- *British Nutrition Foundation*: useful resource relating to food and nutrition providing conference reports, promotes childhood health initiatives – http://www.nutrition.org.uk
- *BSR* (British Society for Rheumatology): rheumatologists' professional body with specialist journal and interest groups – http://www.rheumatology.org.uk
- *Chartered Society of Physiotherapists*: craft society with its own journal – http://www.csp.org.uk
- *European Calcified Tissue Society*: European specialist society offering training courses in osteology and sponsorship of major scientific meetings – http://www.ectsoc.org
- *International Bone and Mineral Society*: international scientific society responsible for major international meetings. Provides practical online resourcing in osteology – http://www.ibmsonline.org
- *International League of Associations for Rheumatism*: professional resource sponsored by the Bone and Joint Decade and Pharmacia – http://www.ilar.org
- *International Society for Clinical Densitometry*: annual scientific meeting, provides educational resources and patient information – http://www.iscd.org
- *National Dairy Council*: promoter of dairy food intake in the UK – http://www.milk.co.uk
- *Royal College of Nursing*: craft society, educational and training resources with strong emphasis on evidence-based practice – http://www.rcn.org.uk
- *Royal College of Obstetricians and Gynaecologists*: professional body providing an educational resource – http://www.rcog.org.uk
- *Royal College of Physicians*: responsible for standard-setting, numerous publications relating to osteoporosis including guidelines for the management of postmenopausal osteoporosis and glucocorticoid-induced osteoporosis – http://www.rcplondon.ac.uk
- *Royal College of Surgeons of England* – http://www.rcseng.ac.uk

GOVERNMENT SITES AND GUIDELINES (UK)

National Institute for Clinical Excellence
11 Strand
London
WC2N 5HR
UK
Tel.: (+44) (0)20 77669 191
Fax: (+44) (0)20 77669123
Website: http://www.nice.org.uk

- *Department of Health* – http://www.doh.gov.uk/osteop.htm
- *Health Development Agency*: identifies the evidence of practices that improve health and reduce health inequality. Supports policy makers and practitioners – http://www.hda-online.org.uk
- *Health Education Board, Scotland*: national agency for health education, health promotion, health advice and health information – http://www.hebs.scot.nhs.uk
- *Health Professions Wales* – http://www.hpw.org.uk
- *NHS Direct online*: provides access to typical illnesses and self-help guide. Advice regarding healthy living and provides information about local databases – http://www.nhsdirect.nhs.uk
- *PRODIGY*: national resource in clinical guidance – research and development and a general resource for all clinicians – http://www.prodigy.nhs.uk

PATIENT AND CARERS' SUPPORT

Age Concern
18 Stephenson Way
London
NW1 2HD
UK
Tel.: (+44) (0)800 009966
Website: http://www.ageconcern.org.uk

ARC (Arthritis Research Campaign)
PO Box 177
Chesterfield
Derbyshire
S41 7TQ
UK
Website: http://www.arc.org.uk

Disabled Living Centres Council
Red Bank House
4 St Chads Street
Manchester
M8 8QA
UK
Tel.: (+44) (0)161 8341044

Royal Association for Disability and Rehabilitation (RADAR)
Unit 12
City Forum
250 City Road
London
EC1V 8AF
UK
Tel.: (+44) (0)20 7250 3222

- Amarant Trust – http://www.amarantmenopausetrust.org.uk
- BackCare – http://www.backpain.org
- British Menopause Society – http://www.the-bms.org
- Brittle Bone Society – http://www.brittlebone.org
- Coeliac Society UK – http://www.coeliac.co.uk
- Disabled Living Foundation – http://www.dlf.org.uk
- Eating Disorders Association – http://www.edauk.com
- Help the Aged – http://www.helptheaged.org.uk
- Telephone Helplines Association – http://www.helplines.org.uk

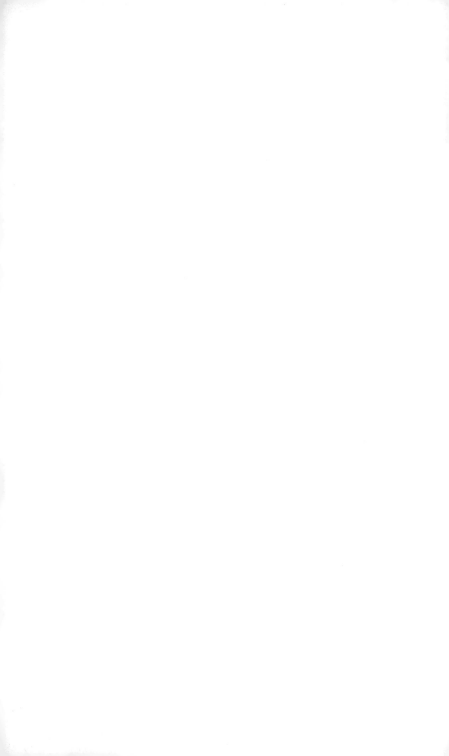

APPENDIX 2
Drugs used to treat osteoporosis

Drug	Trade name	Dose	Regimen	Comments	Common side-effects
Alendronate	Fosamax	10 mg	One tablet taken with a full glass of water on an empty stomach at least 30 minutes before breakfast. Stand or sit upright for at least 30 minutes and avoid lying down until after breakfast. Avoid taking when going to bed or before getting out of bed	Do not take with other medications. Contra-indicated in patients with abnormalities of the oesophagus and other factors which delay emptying	Oesophagitis, abdominal pain, oesophageal ulcers, strictures and erosions have been reported
Alendronate	Fosamax	70 mg	Taken weekly	As above	As above
Etidronate/ calcium	Didronel PMO	400 mg etidronate/ 1000 mg calcium citrate	Take one etidronate tablet daily for 14 days with a large glass of water. Avoid taking food for at least 2 hours before and avoid calcium rich foods or drinks	Do not take with other medications	Abdominal pain and nausea, mainly due to the calcium component of the combined preparation

Drug	Trade name	Dose	Regimen	Comments	Common side-effects
Risedronate	Actonel	5 mg	One tablet taken with a full glass of water on rising or on an empty stomach, at least 30 minutes before food or if taken at other times of the day, 2 hours before or after food, especially avoiding calcium rich food or drinks	Do not take with other treatments. Caution with oesophageal abnormalities and other factors which delay transit or emptying	Upper and lower gastrointestinal side-effects including dyspepsia and diarrhoea
Risedronate	Actonel	35 mg	One tablet weekly	As above	As above
Raloxifene	Evista	60 mg	One tablet daily with or without food	Increases risk of venous thromboembolism. Reduces risk of breast cancer	Muscle cramps, hot flushes
Calcitonin (injectable)	Calsynar, Forcaltonin	100 IU	100 IU per day subcutaneously or intra-muscularly	May have analgesic effect in acute vertebral fracture. Calcium and vitamin D supplements used where advised. Caution with history of allergy	

Drug	Trade name	Dose	Regimen	Comments	Common side-effects
Calcitonin (intranasal)	Miacalcic	200 IU	Take one puff intranasally each day		Rhinitis, epistaxis, headache
Tibolone	Livial	2.5 mg	One tablet daily with or without food	Improves libido and helps menopausal vasomotor symptoms. Do not use until at least one year post-menopause	Hirsutism, deranged liver function tests
Parathyroid hormone (PTH)	Forteo	20 mcg	Daily subcutaneous injection	Synthetic recombinant PTH. Not yet licensed in the UK. Applicability limited by expense and need to self-administer	Nausea, headache and hypercalcaemia
Hormone replacement therapy	Various formu-lations	Various doses	Various regimens	Anti-fracture efficacy attenuated after stopping treatment	Weight gain, fluid retention, breast tenderness, menstrual bleeding; increased risk of breast cancer, ischaemic heart disease and cerebrovascular accident with prolonged use
1,25 Dihydroxy-vitamin D	Rocaltrol	250 ng	1-2 tablets daily	Relatively toxic. Serial monitoring of	Hypercalcaemia

Drug	Trade name	Dose	Regimen	Comments	Common side-effects
Calcium supplements	Various formulations	500–1000 mg	1–2 tablets daily	calcium and renal function advisable Indicated in patients with low dietary calcium; used as an adjunct to other agents in treatment of established osteoporosis	Gastrointestinal upset
Calcium and vitamin D supplements	Various formulations	500–1000 mg calcium; 400–800 IU cholecalciferol	1–2 tablets daily	Indicated in patients with low dietary calcium and vitamin D, and for the primary prevention of fractures in the elderly; used as an adjunct to other agents in treatment of established osteoporosis	Gastrointestinal upset

See Chapter 7 for more detailed comments on the use of these drugs.

REFERENCES

CHAPTER 1

1. World Health Organization 1994 Assessment of fracture risk and its application to screening for post-menopausal osteoporosis. WHO, Geneva, Technical Report Series 843
2. United Nations 1995 The sex and age distribution of populations 1994. Revision of the United Nations global population estimates and projections. United Nations, New York
3. Greendale G A, Barrett-Connor E J, Ingles S et al 1995 Late physical and functional effects of osteoporotic fracture in women: the Rancho Bernardo Study. Journal of the American Geriatric Society 43:955–961
4. National Osteoporosis Society 2002 Primary care strategy for osteoporosis and falls. A framework for health improvement programmes implementing the National Service Framework for Older People. NOS, Bath
5. National Osteoporosis Society 1999 The management of osteoporosis in general practice: results of a national study. Osteoporosis Review 7:1–3
6. Royal College of Physicians 1999 Osteoporosis: clinical guidelines for prevention and treatment. RCP, London
7. Brown P 2001 A five-step management plan for general practice. Osteoporosis Review 9:8–10
8. Department of Health 1998 Quick reference primary care guide on the prevention and treatment of osteoporosis. DOH, London
9. National Osteoporosis Society 1998 Guidance on the prevention and management of corticosteroid induced osteoporosis. NOS, Bath
10. Primary Care Rheumatology Society 1999 Minimum standard guidelines. PCRS, North Allerton, North Yorkshire

CHAPTER 2

1. Cooper C, Melton M J 1992 Epidemiology of osteoporosis. Trends in Epidemiology and Metabolism 3:224–229
2. Doherty D A, Sanders K M, Kotowicz M A, Prince R L 2001 Lifetime and five-year age-specific risks of first and subsequent osteoporotic fractures in postmenopausal women. Osteoporosis International 12(1):16–23
3. Cauley J A, Thompson D E, Ensrud K C et al 2000 Risk of mortality following clinical fractures. Osteoporosis International 11:556–561
4. Royal College of Physicians 1989 Fractured neck of femur. Prevention and management. RCP, London
5. Cummings S R, Nevitt M C 1989 Epidemiology of hip fractures and falls. In: Kleerekoper M, Krane S M (eds) Clinical disorders of bone and mineral metabolism. Mary Ann Liebert, New York, p 231–236
6. Keene G S, Parker M J, Pryor G A 1993 Mortality and morbidity after hip fracture. British Medical Journal 307:1248–1250
7. White B L, Fisher W D, Laurin C A 1987 Rate of mortality for elderly patients after fracture of the hip in the 1980's. Journal of Bone and Joint Surgery 69A:1335–1339

8. Department of Health 1994 Advisory Group on Osteoporosis Report. DOH, London

9. Cooper C, Atkinson E J, Jacobsen S J et al 1993 Population based study of survival after osteoporotic fractures. American Journal of Epidemiology 137:1001–1005

10. Blandy J P 1996 The National Confidential Enquiry into peri-operative deaths. 1993/94 NCEPOD Report. London

11. Campling E A et al 1997 Who operates when. A report by the National Confidential Enquiry into peri-operative deaths. NCEPOD, London

12. Parker M J, Pryor G A 1993 Hip fracture management. Blackwell Scientific, Oxford, p 72–73

13. Chrischilles E A, Butler C D, Davis C S, Wallace R B 1991 Model of lifetime osteoporosis impact. Archives of Internal Medicine 151:2026–2032

14. Cummings S R, Nevitt M C, Browner W S et al 1995 Risk factors for hip fracture in white women. Study of Osteoporotic Fractures Research Group. New England Journal of Medicine 332:767–773

15. Anon. 1998 Osteoporosis: review of the evidence for prevention, diagnosis and treatment and cost effectiveness analysis. Osteoporosis International 8(suppl 4):51–58

16. Wei T S, Hu C H, Wang S H, Hwang K L 2001 Fall characteristics, functional mobility and bone mineral density as risk factors of hip fracture in the community-dwelling ambulatory elderly. Osteoporosis International 12:1050–1055

17. Schurch M A, Rizzoli R, Mermill O D et al 1996 A prospective study on socio-economic aspects of fracture of the proximal femur. Journal of Bone and Mineral Research 11:1935–1942

18. Poor G, Atkinson E J, Lewallen D G et al 1995 Age related hip fracture in men: clinical spectrum and short term outcome. Osteoporosis International 5:419–426

19. Marcus R, Feldman D, Kelsey J (eds) 1996 Age, ethnicity and osteoporosis. In: Osteoporosis. Academic Press, San Diego, p 435–447

20. Spector T S, Cooper C, Lewis A F 1990 Trends in admissions for hip fractures in England and Wales 1968–85. British Medical Journal 300:1173–1174

21. Kanis J A, McCloskey E V 1992 Epidemiology of vertebral osteoporosis. Bone 13:S1–S10

22. Tosteson A N, Gabriel S E, Grove M R 2001 Impact of hip and vertebral fractures on Quality Adjusted Life Years. Osteoporosis International 12:1042–1049

23. O'Neill T, Felsenberg D, Varlow J et al 1996 The European Vertebral Osteoporosis Study Group. The prevalence of vertebral deformity in European men and women. The European Vertebral Osteoporosis Study. Journal of Bone and Mineral Research 11:1010–1018

24. Ross P D, Fujiwara S, Huang C et al 1995 Vertebral fracture prevalence in women in Hiroshima compared to Caucasians or Japanese in the US. International Journal of Epidemiology 24:1171–1177

25. Lau E M, Chan H H, Woo J et al 1996 Normal X-rays for vertebral height ratios and prevalence of vertebral fracture in Hong Kong. Chinese: a comparison with American Caucasians. Journal of Bone and Mineral Research 11:1364–1368

26. Ismail A A, Cooper C, Felsenberg D et al 1999 Number and type of vertebral deformities: epidemiological characteristics and relationship to back pain and height loss. Osteoporosis International 9:206–213

27. Felsenberg D, Lunt M, Ambecht G et al 1994 Rates and determinants of vertebral fracture incidence in European men and women. Journal of Bone and Mineral Research 14:S1105

28. Gibson M J 1987 The prevention of falls in later life. Danish Medical Bulletin 34:(suppl 4):1–24

29. Cuddihy M T, Gabriel S E, Crowson C S et al 1999 Forearm fractures as predictions of subsequent osteoporotic fractures. Osteoporosis International 9(6):469–475

30. Kaukonen J P, Karaharjh E O, Porras M et al 1998 Functional recovery after fractures of the distal forearm. Annales Chirurgiae et Gynaecologiae 77:27–31

CHAPTER 3

1. Barker D J P (ed) 1994 Programming the baby. In: Mothers, babies and disease in later life. BMJ Publishing, London, p 14–36

2. Smith D M, Nance W E, Kang K W et al 1973 Genetic factors in determining bone mass. Journal of Clinical Investigation 52:2800–2808

3. Pocock N, Eisman J A, Hopper J L et al 1987 Genetic determinants of bone mass in adults. A twin study. Journal of Clinical Investigation 80:706–710

4. Melton L J 1991 Differing patterns of osteoporosis across the world. In: Chesnut C H (ed) New dimensions in osteoporosis in the 1990's. Excerpta Medica, Hong Kong, p 13–18

5. Cummings S R, Nevitt M C 1989 Epidemiology of hip fractures and falls. In: Kleerekoper M, Krane S M (eds) Clinical disorders of bone and mineral metabolism. Mary Ann Liebert, New York, p 231–236

6. Matkovic V, Fontana D, Tominac C et al 1990 Factors that influence peak bone mass formation – a study of calcium balance and the inheritance of bone mass in adolescent females. American Journal of Clinical Nutrition 52:878–888

7. Johnston C C, Millar J Z, Siemenda C W et al 1992 Calcium supplementation and increases in bone mineral density in children. New England Journal of Medicine 327:82–87

8. Lloyd T, Andon M, Rollings N et al 1993 Calcium supplementation and bone mineral density in adolescent girls. Journal of the American Medical Association 270:841–844

9. Lee W T K, Leung S S F, Lui S S H et al 1994 Double blind, controlled calcium supplementation and bone mineral accretion in children accustomed to a low calcium diet. American Journal of Clinical Nutrition 60:744–750

10. Nowson C A, Green R M, Hopper J L et al 1997 A co-twin study of the effect of calcium supplementation on bone density during adolescence. Osteoporosis International 7:219–225

11. Slemenda C W, Miller J Z, Hui S L et al 1991 Role of physical activity in the development of skeletal mass in children. Journal of Bone and Mineral Research 6:1227–1233

12. Ruiz J C, Mandel C, Garpibedian M 1995 Influence of spontaneous calcium intake and physical exercise on the vertebral and femoral bone mineral density of children and adolescents. Journal of Bone and Mineral Research 10:675–682

13. Garwero P, Hausherr E, Chapuy M C et al 1996 Markers of bone resorption predict hip fracture in elderly women: the EPIDOS study. Journal of Bone and Mineral Research 11:1531–1538

14. Riggs B L, Wahner W, Seeman E et al 1982 Changes in bone mineral density of the proximal femur and spine with

ageing: differences between the post-menopausal and senile osteoporotic syndromes. Journal of Clinical Investigation 70:716–723

15. Dresner-Pollak R, Parker R A, Poku M et al 1996 Biochemical markers of bone turnover reflect femoral bone loss in elderly women. Calcified Tissue International 59:328–333

16. Slemenda C W, Longcope C, Zhow L et al 1997 Sex steroids and bone mass in older men: positive associations with serum estrogens and negative associations with androgens. Journal of Clinical Investigation 100:1755–1759

17. Greendale S A, Edelstein S, Barrett-Connor E 1997 Endogenous sex steroids and bone mineral density in older women and men: The Rancho-Bernardo Study. Journal of Bone and Mineral Research 121:1833–1843

18. Law M R, Hackshaw A K 1997 A meta analysis of cigarette smoking, bone mineral density and risk of hip fracture: recognition of a major effect. British Medical Journal 315:841–846

19. Seeman E 1996 The effect of tobacco and alcohol use in bone. In: Marcus R, Feldman D, Kelsey J (eds) Osteoporosis. Academic Press, San Diego, p 373–393

20. Horowitz M C 1993 Cytokines and oestrogen in bone: anti-osteoporotic effects. Science 260:626–627

21. Jilka R L 1998 Cytokines, bone remodelling and oestrogen deficiency; 1998 update. Bone 23:75–81

CHAPTER 4

1. Cooper C, Melton L J 1992 Vertebral fractures: how large is the silent epidemic? British Medical Journal 304:793 –794

2. Royal College of Physicians 1999 Osteoporosis: clinical guidelines for prevention and treatment. RCP, London

3. Cummings S R, Nevitt M C, Browner W S et al 1995 Risk factors for hip fracture in white women. Study of Osteoporotic Fractures Research Group. New England Journal of Medicine 332:767–773

4. Melton L J, Kan S H, Frye M A et al 1989 Epidemiology of vertebral fractures in women. American Journal of Epidemiology 129:1000–1011

5. Nguygen T, Sambrook P, Kelly P et al 1993 Predictors of osteoporotic fractures by postural instability and bone density. British Medical Journal 307:1111–1115

6. Francis R M, Peacock M, Marshall D H et al 1989 Spinal osteoporosis in men. Journal of Bone and Mineral Research 5:347–357

7. Baillie S P, Davison C E, Johnson F J, Francis R M 1992 Pathogenesis of vertebral crush fractures in men. Age and Ageing 21:139–141

8. McLellan A R, Fraser M, Brown J, O'Brien P J 2000 The osteoporosis/orthopaedics liaison nurse: a model for effecting secondary prevention of osteoporotic fractures in an orthopaedic and accident and emergency setting. Journal of Bone and Mineral Research 15(suppl 1):S439

9. McLellan A R, Fraser M 2002 The fracture liaison service. Osteoporosis Review 10:8–10

10. Scane A C, Francis R M, Sutcliffe A M et al 1999 Case control study of the pathogenesis and sequelae of symptomatic vertebral fractures in men. Osteoporosis International 9:91–97

11. Selby P L, Davies M, Adams JE 2000 Do men and women fracture bones at similar bone densities? Osteoporosis International 11:153–157

12. Smith R, Athanasou N A, Ostlere S J, Vipond S E 1995 Pregnancy associated osteoporosis. Quarterly Journal of Medicine 88:865–878

CHAPTER 5

1. Cooper C, Aihie A 1994 Osteoporosis: recent advances in pathogenesis and treatment. Quarterly Journal of Medicine 87: 203–209

2. Marshall D, Johnell O, Wedel H 1996 Meta-analysis of how well measurements of bone density predict occurrence of osteoporotic fracture. British Medical Journal 312:1254–1259

3. Hans D, Dargent-Molina P, Schott A M et al 1996 Ultrasonographic heel measurements to predict hip fractures in elderly women: the EPIDOS prospective study. Lancet 348:511–514

4. Cummings S R, Nevitt M C, Browner W C et al 1995 Risk factors for hip fracture in white women. Study of Osteoporotic Fractures Research Group. New England Journal of Medicine 332:767–773

5. Jones T, Davie M J 1998 Bone mineral density at distal forearm can identify patients with osteoporosis at the spine or femoral neck. British Journal of Rheumatology 37:539–543

6. Liberman V A, Weiss S R, Broll J, Minne H W Effect of oral alendronate on bone mineral density and the incidence of fractures in post menopausal osteoporosis. New England Journal of Medicine 333:1437–1443

7. Department of Health 2000 The Ionising Radiation Regulations 1999. Statutory instrument 1999, Number 3232. The Stationery Office, London

8. Department of Health 2000 The Ionising Radiation (Medical exposure) Regulations 2000. Statutory instrument 2000, Number 1059. The Stationery Office, London

9. National Osteoporosis Society 2001 Position statement on the use of peripheral X-ray absorptiometry in the management of osteoporosis. NOS, Bath

10. Bauer D C, Gluer C C, Cauley J A et al 1997 Broadband ultrasound attenuation predicts fractures strongly and independently of densitometry in older women. A prospective study. Study of Osteoporotic Fractures Research Group. Archives of Internal Medicine 157:629–634

11. Duppe H, Gardsell P, Nilsson B, Johnell O 1997 A single bone density measurement can predict fractures over 25 years. Calcified Tissue International 60:171–174

12. Nicholson P H, Muller R, Lowet G et al 1998 Do quantitative ultrasound measurements reflect structure independently of density in human cancellous bones? Bone 23:425–431

13. Bouxsein M L, Radloff S E 1997 Quantitative ultrasound reflects the mechanical properties of calcaneal trabeculous bone. Journal of Bone and Mineral Research 12:839–846

14. National Osteoporosis Society 2001 Position statement on the use of quantitative ultrasound in the management of osteoporosis. NOS, Bath

15. Langton C M, Ballard P A, Bennett D K, Purdie D W 1997 Maximising the cost effectiveness of BMD referral for DXA using ultrasound as a selective population pre-screen. Technology in Healthcare 5: 235–241

16. Stewart A, Reid D M 2000 Quantitative ultrasound or clinic risk factors – which identifies women at risk of osteoporosis? British Journal of Radiology 73:165–171

17. Eastell R, Price C P (eds) 1998 Biochemical markers of bone turnover. Supraregional Assay Service. PRU Publications, Sheffield

18. Eastell R, Bainbridge P 2001 Bone turnover markers for monitoring anti-resorptive therapy. Osteoporosis Review 9:1–5

CHAPTER 6

1. Dolan P, Torgerson D J 1998 The costs of treating osteoporotic fractures in the UK female population. Osteoporosis International 8:611–617

2. Writing Group for the Women's Health Initiative Investigators 2002 Risks and benefits of oestrogen plus progestogen in healthy post-menopausal women. Journal of the American Medical Association 288:321–323

3. Compston J E, Cooper C, Kanis J A 1995 Bone densitometry in clinical practice. British Medical Journal 310:1507–1510

4. Ettinger B, Grady D 1994 Maximising the benefit of oestrogen therapy for prevention of osteoporosis. Menopause 1:19–24

5. National Osteoporosis Society 2002 Primary care strategy for osteoporosis and falls. A framework for health improvement programmes implementing the National Service Framework for Older People. NOS, Bath

6. Cauley J A, Lucas F L, Kuller L H et al 1996 Bone mineral density and risk of breast cancer in older women. Journal of the American Medical Association 276:1404–1408

7. Eddy D M, Johnston C C, Cummings S R et al 1998 Osteoporosis: cost effectiveness analysis and review of the evidence for prevention, diagnosis and treatment. Osteoporosis International Suppl 4

8. Cummings S R, Black D M, Thompson D E et al 1998 Effect of alendronate on risk of fracture in women with low bone density but without fractures. Journal of the American Medical Association 280:2077–2082

9. Kanis J A, Brazier J, Calvert N et al 2001 Treatment of established osteoporosis. A report for the NHS Research and Development Health Technology Assessment Programme. Department of Health, London

10. Royal College of Physicians 1999 Osteoporosis: clinical guidelines for prevention and treatment. RCP, London

CHAPTER 7

1. Ralston S H 1997 Osteoporosis. British Medical Journal 315:469–472

2. Department of Health 1998 Committee on medical aspects of food and nutrition policy (COMA). DOH, London

3. Morris F L, Naughton S A, Gibbs J L et al 1997 Prospective ten month exercise intervention in pre-menarcheal girls – positive effects on bone and lean mass. Journal of Bone and Mineral Research 12:1453–1462

4. Wolff I, Van Croonenborg J J, Kemper H C G et al 1999 The effect of exercise training programs on bone mass: a meta analysis of published controlled trials in pre- and post-menopausal women. Osteoporosis International 9:1–12

5. Heinonen A, McKay H, Whithall K et al 2000 Muscle volume is associated with specific site of bone in pre-pubertal girls: a quantitative MR study. Special pre ASBMR meeting on paediatric bone. Exercise and nutrition as modulating factors in skeletal development of children in health and disease. Journal of Bone and Mineral Research 25(suppl 1):300

6. Kannos P, Haapasalo H, Sankelo M et al 1995 Effect of starting age of physical activity on bone mass in the dominant arm of tennis and squash players. Annals of Internal Medicine 123(1):27–31

7. Bradney M, Pearce G, Naughton G et al 1998 Moderate exercise during

growth in prepubertal boys. Changes in bone mass, size, volumetric density and bone strength: a controlled prospective study. Journal of Bone and Mineral Research 13(12):1814–1821

8. Keen A, Drinkwater B 1997 Irreversible bone loss in former amenorrhoeic athletes. Osteoporosis International 7:311–315

9. Reid I R, Legge M, Stapleton J P 1995 Regular exercise dissociates fat mass and bone density in premenopausal women. Journal of Clinical Endocrinology and Metabolism 80:1764–1768

10. Royal College of Physicians 1999 Osteoporosis: clinical guidelines for prevention and treatment. RCP, London

11. Kanis J A 1994 Calcium nutrition and its implications for osteoporosis. Parts I and II. European Journal of Clinical Nutrition 48:757–767, 833–841

12. Recker R R, Kimmel P B, Hinders S et al 1994 Anti-fracture efficacy of calcium in elderly women. Journal of Bone and Mineral Research 9(suppl 1):S154

13. Reid I R, Ames R W, Evans M C et al 1993 Effects of calcium supplementation on bone loss in post-menopausal women. New England Journal of Medicine 328:460–464

14. Chevalley T, Rizzoli R, Nydeggar V et al 1994 Effects of calcium supplements on female bone mineral density and vertebral fracture rate in vitamin D replete elderly patients. Osteoporosis International 4:245–252

15. Kanis J A, Johnell O, Gullberg B et al 1992 Evidence for the efficacy of bone active drugs in the prevention of hip fracture. British Medical Journal 305:1124–1128

16. Chapuy M C, Arlot M E, Du Boef F et al 1992 Vitamin D3 and calcium to prevent hip fractures in elderly women. New England Journal of Medicine 27:1637–1641

17. Lips P, Graafmans W C, Ooms M E et al 1996 Vitamin D supplementation and fracture incidence in elderly persons – a randomised placebo-controlled clinical trial. Annals of Internal Medicine 124:400–406

18. Heikinheimo R J, Inkovaara J A, Harju E J et al 1992 Annual injection of vitamin D and fractures of aged bones. Calcified Tissue International 51:105–110

19. Dawson-Hughes B, Harris S S, Krall E A 1997 Effect of calcium and vitamin D supplementation on bone density in men and women 65 years of age and older. New England Journal of Medicine 337:670–676

20. Cummings S R, Nevitt M C, Browner W S et al 1995 Risk factors for hip fracture in white women. Study of Osteoporotic Fractures Research Group. New England Journal of Medicine 332:767–773

21. Feder G, Cryer C, Donovan S et al 2000 Guidelines for the prevention of falls in people over 65. The Guidelines Development Group. British Medical Journal 321:1007–1011

22. Simey P, Pennington B 1994 Physical activity and the prevention and management of falls and accidents in older people: guidelines for practice. Health Education Authority, London

23. Lindsay R, Hart D M, Forrest C et al 1980 Prevention of spinal osteoporosis in oophorectomised women. Lancet ii:1151–1153

24. Lufkin E G, Wahner H W, O'Fallen W M et al 1992 Treatment of post-menopausal osteoporosis with transdermal oestrogen. Annals of Internal Medicine 117:1–9

25. Hulley S, Grady D, Bush T et al 1998 Randomised trial of estrogen plus progestogen for secondary prevention

of coronary heart disease in post-menopausal women. Journal of the American Medical Association 280:605–613

26. Lacey J V, Mink P J, Lubin J H et al 2002 Menopausal hormone replacement therapy and the risk of ovarian cancer. Journal of the American Medical Association 288:334–341

27. Committee on Safety of Medicines and Medicines Control Agency 2002 Possible risks associated with using HRT. Current Problems in Pharmacovigilance, vol. 28

28. Writing Group for the Women's Health Initiative Investigators 2002 Risks and benefits of oestrogen plus progestogen in healthy post-menopausal women. Journal of the American Medical Association 288:321–323

29. Grady D, Herrington D, Bittner V et al 2002 Cardiovascular disease outcomes during 6.8 years of hormone therapy: Heart and Estrogen/progestin Replacement Study follow-up (HERS II). Journal of the American Medical Association 228:49–57

30. Michaelsson K, Baron JA, Farahamand B et al 1998 Hormone replacement therapy and risk of hip fracture; population based case control study. The Swedish Hip Fracture Study Group. British Medical Journal 316:1858–1863

31. Dupont W D, Page D L, Parl F F et al 1999 Estrogen replacement therapy in women with a history of proliferative breast disease. Cancer 85:1277–1283

32. Barret-Connor E, Grady D, Sashegyi A et al 2002 Raloxifene and cardiovascular events in osteoporotic post-menopausal women – 4 year results from the MORE (Multiple Outcomes of Raloxifene Evaluation)

randomised trial. Journal of the American Medical Association 287:847–857

33. Cauley J, Norton L, Lippman M et al 2001 Continued breast cancer reduction in post-menopausal women treated with raloxifene: 4 year results from the MORE trial. Breast Cancer Research and Treatment 65:125–134

34. Delmas P D, Bjarnason N H, Mitlak B H et al 1997 Effects of Raloxifene on bone mineral density, serum cholesterol concentrations and uterine endometrium in post-menopausal women. New England Journal of Medicine 337:1641–1647

35. Ettinger B, Black D M, Mitlak B H et al 1999 Reduction of vertebral fracture risk in post-menopausal women with osteoporosis treated with Raloxifene. Results from a 3 year randomised clinical trial. Journal of the American Medical Association 282:637–645

36. Hosking D, Chilvers C E D, Christiansen C et al 1998 Prevention of bone loss with Alendronate in post-menopausal women under 60 years of age. New England Journal of Medicine 338:485–492

37. Chesnut C H, McClung M R, Ensrud K E et al 1995 Alendronate treatment of the post-menopausal osteoporotic woman: effect of multiple dosages on bone mass and bone remodelling. American Journal of Medicine 99:144–152

38. Black D M, Cummings S R, Karpf D B et al 1997 Randomised trial of effect of Alendronate on risk of fracture in women with existing vertebral fractures. Lancet 348:1535–1541

39. Cummings S R, Black D M, Thompson D E et al 1998 Effect of Alendronate on risk of fracture in women with low bone density but without vertebral fractures – results

from the Fracture Intervention Trial. Journal of the American Medical Association 280:2077–2082

40. Pols H A, Felsenberg D, Hanley D A et al 1999 Multinational placebo controlled randomised trial of the effects of Alendronate on bone density and fracture risk in post-menopausal women with low bone mass: results of the FOSIT study. Osteoporosis International 9:461–468

41. Schnitzer T, Bone H G, Crepaldi G et al 2000 Therapeutic equivalence of alendronate 70 mg weekly and alendronate 10 mg daily in the treatment of osteoporosis. Aging, Clinical and Experimental Research 12:1–12

42. Storm T, Thamsborg G, Steiniche T et al 1990 Effect of intermittent cyclical Etidronate therapy on bone mass and fracture rate in women with post-menopausal osteoporosis. New England Journal of Medicine 322:1265–1271

43. Watts N, Harris S T, Genant H K et al 1990 Intermittent cyclical etidronate treatment of postmenopausal osteoporosis. New England Journal of Medicine 323:73–79

44. Harris S T, Watts N B, Jackson R D et al 1993 Four-year study of intermittent cyclical etidronate treatment of postmenopausal osteoporosis: three years of blinded therapy followed by one year of open therapy. American Journal of Medicine 95:557–567

45. Herd R J, Balena R, Blake G H et al 1997 Prevention of early post-menopausal bone loss by cyclical Etidronate: a two year double-blind placebo controlled study. American Journal of Medicine 103:92–99

46. Van Staa T D, Abenhaim L, Cooper C et al 1998 Use of cyclical Etidronate and prevention of new vertebral fractures. British Journal of Rheumatology 37:87–94

47. Harris S T, Watts N B, Genant H K et al 1999 Effects of Risedronate treatment on vertebral and non-vertebral fractures in women with post-menopausal osteoporosis. A randomised controlled trial. Journal of the American Medical Association 282:1344–1352

48. Reginster J-Y, Minne H W, Sorensen O H et al 2000 Randomised trial of the effects of Risedronate on vertebral fractures in women with established post-menopausal osteoporosis. Osteoporosis International 11:83–91

49. Geusens P, Adami S, Bensen W et al 2000 Risedronate reduces risk of hip fractures in elderly women with osteoporosis. Calcified Tissue International 66:56 (abstract)

50. Chesnut C H III, Silverman S, Andriano K et al 2000 A randomised trial of nasal spray salmon calcitonin in post-menopausal women with established osteoporosis: the prevention of recurrence of osteoporotic fractures study. American Journal of Medicine 109:267–276

51. Kanis J A, McCloskey E V 1999 The effect of calcitonin on vertebral and other fractures. Quarterly Journal of Medicine 92:143–149

52. Lyritis G P, Tsakalakos N, Magiasis B et al 1991 Analgesic effect of salmon calcitonin in osteoporotic vertebral fractures: a double blind placebo controlled clinical study. Calcified Tissue International 49:369–372

53. Tilyard M W, Spears G F, Thomson J et al 1992 Treatment of post-menopausal osteoporosis with calcitriol or calcium. New England Journal of Medicine 326:357–362

54. Gallagher J C, Riggs B L, Recker R R, Goldgar D 1989 The effect of calcitriol

on patients with postmenopausal osteoporosis with special reference to fracture frequency. Proceedings of the Society for Experimental Biology and Medicine 191:287–292

55. Neer R M, Arnaud C, Zanchetta J R et al 2001 Effect of parathyroid hormone (1-34) on fractures and bone mineral density in postmenopausal women with osteoporosis. New England Journal of Medicine 344:1434–1441

56. Rittmaster R S, Bolognese M, Ettinger M P et al 2000 Enhancement of bone mass in osteoporotic women with parathyroid hormone followed by Alendronate. Journal of Clinical Endocrinology and Metabolism 85:2129–2134

CHAPTER 8

1. Anderson F H, Francis R M, Bishop J C et al 1997 Effect of intermittent etidronate therapy on bone mineral density in men with vertebral fractures. Age & Ageing 26:359–365

2. Ho Y V, Frauman A S, Thomson W et al 2000 Effects of alendronate on bone density in men with primary and secondary osteoporosis. Osteoporosis International 11:98–101

3. Orwoll C, Ettinger M, Weiss S et al 2000 Alendronate for the treatment of osteoporosis in men. New England Journal of Medicine 343:604–610

4. Van Staa T P, Leulkens H, Abenhaim L et al 2000 The use of oral corticosteroids and the risk of fractures. Journal of Bone and Mineral Research 15(6):993–1000

5. Eastell R, Boyle I T, Compston J et al 1998 Management of male osteoporosis. Report of the UK Concensus Group. Quarterly Journal of Medicine 91:71–92

6. Behre H M, Von Eckardstein S, Kliesh S et al 1999 Long term substitution therapy of hypogonadal men with transcrotal testosterone over 7–10 years. Clinical Endocrinology 50:629–635

7. Orwoll E S, Oviatt S K, McClung M R et al 1990 The rate of bone loss in normal men and the effects of calcium and cholecalciferol supplementation. Annals of Internal Medicine 112:29–34

8. Dawson-Hughes B, Harris S S, Krall E A 1997 Effect of calcium and vitamin D supplementation on bone density in men and women 65 years of age and older. New England Journal of Medicine 337:670–676

9. Heikinhomo R J, Inkovaara J A, Harju E J et al 1992 Annual injection of vitamin D and fractures of aged bone. Calcified Tissue International 55:105–110

10. Van Staa T P, Leulkens H G, Abenhaim L et al 2000 Use of oral corticosteroids in the UK. Quarterly Journal of Medicine 93:105–111

11. Van Staa T P, Leulkens HG, Cooper C 2001 Use of inhaled corticosteroids and risk of fractures. Journal of Bone and Mineral Research 16(3):581–588

12. Royal College of Physicians 2003 Guidelines on the prevention and treatment of glucocorticoid induced osteoporosis. RCP, London

13. Van Staa T P, Abenhaim L, Cooper C et al 2001 Public health impact of adverse bone effects of oral corticosteroids. British Journal of Clinical Pharmacology 51:601–607

14. American College of Sports Medicine 1997 Position stand on the female athletic triad. Medicine and Science in Sports and Exercise 29:i–ix

15. Bennell K L, Malcolm S A, Wark J D et al 1997 Skeletal effects of menstrual disturbances in athletes. Scandinavian Journal of Medicine and Science in Sports 7:261–273

16. Carmichael K A, Carmichael D H 1995 Bone metabolism and osteopenia in eating disorders. Medicine 74:254–267

17. Klibanski A, Biller B M K, Schoenfeld D A et al 1995 The effects of oestrogen administration on trabecular bone loss in young women with anorexia nervosa. Journal of Clinical Endocrinology and Metabolism 80:898–904

CHAPTER 9

1. Gennari C, Agnusdei D, Camporeale A 1991 Use of calcitonin in the treatment of bone pain associated with osteoporosis. Calcified Tissue International 49(suppl 2):S9–13

2. Tolini A, Romano L, Ronsini S et al 1993 Treatment of post menopausal osteoporosis with salmon calcitonin nasal spray: evaluation by bone mineral content and biochemical patterns. International Journal of Clinical Pharmacology and Therapeutic Toxicology 31:358–360

3. Abellan Perez M, Bayina Garcia F J, Calabozo M et al 1995 Multicenter comparative study of synthetic salmon calcitonin administered nasally in the treatment of established post menopausal osteoporosis. Anales de Medicina Interna 12:12–16

4. Hall J, Skevington M, Maddison P J et al 1996 A randomised controlled trial of hydrotherapy in rheumatoid arthritis. Arthritis Care and Research 3:206–215

5. Braud L J, Cauthier P, Rox P M et al 1997 A weight bearing water based exercising programme for osteopenic women: its impact on bone fracture and well being. Archives of Physical Medicine and Rehabilitation 78(12):1375–1380

6. Lord S R, Ward J A, Williams P et al 1995 The effect of a 12 month exercise trial on balance, strength and falls in older women: a randomised controlled trial. Journal of the American Geriatrics Society 43:1198–1206

CHAPTER 10

1. Tinetti M E, Speechley M, Ginter S F 1988 Risk factors for falls among elderly persons living in the community. New England Journal of Medicine 319:1701–1707

2. Campbell A J, Reinken J, Allan B C et al 1981 Falls in old age: a study of frequency and related clinical factors. Age and Ageing 10:264–270

3. Lord S R, McClean D, Stathers S 1992 Physiological factors associated with injurious fall in older people living in the community. Gerentology 38:338–346

4. Department of Trade and Industry 1998 Avoiding slips, trips and broken hips. Accidental falls in the home; Regional distribution of people over 65 in the UK. DTI, London

5. Kanis J A 1996 Textbook of osteoporosis. Blackwell Scientific, Oxford, p 133

6. Lauritzen J B 1997 Hip fractures, epidemiology, risk factors, falls energy absorption, hip protectors and prevention. Danish Medical Bulletin 44:155–168

7. Lord S R, Ward J A 1994 Age associated differences in sensori-motor function and balance in community dwelling women. Age and Ageing 23:452–460

8. Snow Harter C, Bouxsein M, Lewis B et al 1990 Muscle strength as a predictor of bone mineral density in young women. Journal of Bone and Mineral Research 5:589–595

9. Pocock N, Eisman J, Gwinn T et al 1989 Muscle strength, physical fitness and weight but not age predicted

femoral neck bone mass. Journal of Bone and Mineral Research 4:441–448

10. Kritz-Silverstein D, Barret-Connor E 1994 Grip strength and bone mineral density in older women. Journal of Bone and Mineral Research 9:45–51

11. Lord S R, Ward J A, Williams P et al 1995 The effect of a 12 minute exercise trial on balance, strength and falls in older women: a randomised controlled trial. Journal of the American Geriatrics Society 43:1198–1206

12. Pfeifer M, Begerow W, Minne H W et al 2000 Effects of short term vitamin D and calcium supplementation on body sway and secondary hyperparathyroidism in elderly women. Journal of Bone and Mineral Research 15:1113–1118

13. Masud T 2002 Fall prevention in osteoporosis. Osteoporosis Review 3:9–12

14. Close J, Ellis M, Hooper R et al 1999 Prevention of falls in the elderly trial (PROFET): a randomised controlled trial. Lancet 353:93–97

15. Tinetti M E, Baker D I, McAvay G et al 1994 A multifactoral intervention to reduce the risk of falling amongst elderly people living in the community. New England Journal of Medicine 331:821–827

16. Lauritzen J B, Petersen M M, Lund B 1993 Effect of external hip protectors on hip fractures. Lancet 341:11–13

17. American Geriatrics Society, British Geriatrics Society and American Academy of Orthopaedic Surgeons Panel on fall prevention 2001 Guidelines for the prevention of falls in older persons. Journal of the American Geriatrics Society 49:664–672

18. Department of Health 2001 National Service Framework for older people. The Stationery Office, London

19. National Osteoporosis Society 2002 Primary care strategy for osteoporosis and falls. A framework for health improvement programmes implementing the National Service Framework for older people. NOS, Bath

CHAPTER 11

1. Consensus Development Conference 2001 Journal of the American Medical Association 285:785–795

2. Royal College of Physicians 1999 Osteoporosis: clinical guidelines for prevention and treatment. RCP, London

3. Cummings S R, Nevitt M C, Browner W S et al 1995 Risk factors for hip fracture in white women. Study of Osteoporotic Fractures Research Group. New England Journal of Medicine 332:767–773

4. Department of Health 2001 National Service Framework for older people. The Stationery Office, London

GLOSSARY OF ACRONYMS

BBUA – broadband ultrasonic attenuation

BMC – bone mineral content

BMD – bone mineral density

BMI – body mass index

CEE – conjugated equine estrogen

COMA – (Department of Health) Committee on medical aspects of food and nutrition policy

COPD – chronic obstructive pulmonary disease

CVA – cerebrovascular accident

DHS – dynamic hip screw

DXA – dual energy X-ray absorptiometry

EPIDOS – Epidemiology of Osteoporosis Study

EVOS – European Vertebral Osteoporosis Study

FIT – Fracture Intervention Trial

FSH – follicle stimulating hormone

GIO – glucocorticoid-induced osteoporosis

GPRD – General Practice Research Database

HERS – heart and estrogen/progestin replacement study

HRT – hormone replacement therapy

IHD – ischaemic heart disease

IL1 – interleukin 1

IL6 – interleukin 6

LFR – lifetime fracture risk

LH – luteinising hormone

MORE – multiple outcomes of raloxifene evaluation

MRI – magnetic resonance imaging

NHANES – National Health and Nutrition Examination Survey

NOS – National Osteoporosis Society

PCO – primary care organisation

pDXA – peripheral DXA

PMO – postmenopausal osteoporosis

PSA – prostate specific antigen

PTH – parathyroid hormone

QALY – quality adjusted life year(s)

QCT – quantitative computed tomography

QUI – qualitative ultrasound index

QUS – quantitative ultrasound

RCTs – randomised controlled trials

RR – relative risk

SERM – selective (o)estrogen receptor modulator

SHBG – sex hormone binding globulin

SIP – sickness impact profile

SOF – Study of Osteoporotic Fractures

SOS – speed of sound

STIR – short tau inversion recovery

TSH – thyroid stimulating hormone

TNFα – tumour necrosis factor α

TNS – transcutaneous nerve stimulation

WHI – Women's Health Initiative

WHO – World Health Organization

LIST OF PATIENT QUESTIONS

INDEX

Note: Numbers in **bold** refer to boxes/figures/tables

A

Abdominal distension, 28
Absolute risk assessment, 178
Acronyms (listed), 205
Activation frequency, 46
Acupuncture, pain management using, 40, **159**
Afro-Caribbean subjects
  incidence of hip fractures, 26, **27**
  osteoporotic fracture rates, 49
  risk of osteoporosis, 58
  vertebral deformity, 32
Age Concern, address and website, 186
Age-related decline of bone density, **3–4**, 58
Age-related decline of cognitive function, and risk of falls, **168**, 170
Age-related hormone levels, 54
Age-related incidence rates, fractures, 15, **16**, 35, 37, 63
Age-related prevalence of osteoporosis, **6**
Alcohol
  effect on bone density, 60, 136
  maximal intake advised, 136
Alcohol (excess) intake
  bone mass/density/strength affected by, 54, 117
  effect on incidence of hip fracture, **19**
  gender differences, 18
  reduction of, and bone loss, **112**
  as risk factor for osteoporosis, 54, 58, 60, 117, 136
  and risk of falls, **19**, 24, **169**, 170
Alcoholics
  presentation of osteoporosis, 54, 60
  testosterone levels, 54, 58
Alcoholism, effects, **19**
Alendronate, 126–127, 189
  anti-fracture efficacy, **126**, 126–127, 179
  contraindications, 189
  cost effectiveness, **102**, 103
  dosage, 126, 189
  effect on bone loss, **112**
  effect on bone mineral density, 126
  osteoporosis treated with, **118**
    in men, 139, 143, 153
  prescribing in general practice, **9**
  side-effects, 189

  steroid-induced osteoporosis treated with, **149**
  weekly dosing, 127, 128
Alfacalcidol, 131, 140, **149**
Algodystrophy (reflex sympathetic dystrophy), 35, 41, 158
  in children, **72**
Amarant Trust, 187
  literature on HRT, 138
Amenorrhoea, and osteoporosis, 50, 51, 112, 151
American Society for Bone and Mineral Research, 184
  case-finding approach to prevention, 62
Anabolic agents
  future developments, 179
  osteoporosis treated using, **118**, 131–132, 144, 151
  side-effects, 131, 132
Analgesics
  for pain control, 40, 158, **159**
  prescribing in general practice, **9**
  side-effects, 40
Anorexia, and osteoporosis, 51, 54, 111, 151
Anorexics, treatment of, 151
Anticonvulsants
  and fracture risk, **19**, 24
  and osteoporosis, **19**, **72**, 117, 152
Antidepressants
  in rehabilitation after fracture, **159**, 160, 161
  and risk of falls, **19**, **168**
Anti-resorptives, osteoporosis treated with, 117–118, 138
Apposition, 47
Arthralgia, as side-effect, 131
Arthritis
  juvenile, as cause of osteoporosis, **72**, 151
  and risk of falls, **19**, **168**, 170
Arthritis Research Campaign (ARC), address and website, 186
Asian subjects
  incidence of hip fractures, 26, **27**
  osteoporotic fracture rates, 49
  risk of osteoporosis, 58
  vertebral deformity, 32
Asymptomatic osteoporosis, 2, 11, 64
Atherosclerosis (hardening of arteries), 137, 138
Athletes with amenorrhoea, and osteoporosis, 50, 51, 112, 151, 155

I

X

Z

W